Remarkable Journey

Breast Implant Illness and Cancer

Roann & Jim,
People who knew
my through my
Amazing & Remarkable
Journey
Deborah
Nottingham

Deborah Nottingham

Published 2020
Published by KPN
ISBN 978-1-7353848-0-1 Paperback
ISBN 978-1-7353848-1-8 Kindle

Library of Congress Control Number 2020912622

Written by Deborah Nottingham
Cover Design by Debra Phillips AdExcellence.net
Cover Art by © Can Stock Photo Inc. / focalpoint

Editing by Debra L. Butterfield

Medical disclaimer: This medical information is merely information — not advice. If users need medical advice, they should consult a doctor or other appropriate medical professional. The disclaimer provides no warranties in relation to the medical information supplied on any website, and that no liability will accrue to the author in the event that a user suffers loss as a result of reliance upon the information.

Every effort has been made to ensure that all the information in this book is accurate at the time of publication; however, the author neither endorses nor guarantees the content of external links referenced in this book.

Printed in the United States of America

Author Biography

Deborah Nottingham loves to travel and went to China to ride elephants for her sixtieth birthday after riding camels in Egypt for her fiftieth birthday. She loves to hike, especially in Colorado, and has hiked in all 50 states and many countries. She is a graduate of Indiana University with a BS in Medical Technology, and the University of Houston with an MBA. Her corporate career was in healthcare in sales and marketing for thirty years. Debi and her husband owned an escape room for five years.

Note from the Author:

Reviews are gold to authors! If you have enjoyed this book, would you consider reviewing it on Amazon.com or GoodReads?

Other Books by Deborah Nottingham *Deception: Revelation to Release Response to My Christian Gay Spouse* http://covenantbooks.com/books/?book=deception-revelation-to-release

Read more from Deborah Nottingham at http://Debdays.wordpress.com

Join her email list at http://DeborahNottingham.com

Debi can be reached at Debidays@gmail.com

Contents

To die is nothing; but it is terrible not to live.
—Victor Hugo, *Les Misérables*

What began the change was the very writing itself...
Memory once waked will play the tyrant...
The change which the writing wrought in me was only a beginning
—only to prepare me for the gods' surgery.
They used my own pen to probe my wound.
—C. S. Lewis, *Till We Have Faces*

Hope has two beautiful daughters; their names are anger and courage.
Anger that things are the way they are.
Courage to make them the way they ought to be.
—St. Augustine

Chapter 1

It Started with a Horse

My journey of breast implant illness started with a horse. The horse bucked and off I went, tumbling through the air. I landed with a thud on my right side. My fingers were jammed and I couldn't catch my breath as my shoulder and neck were jerked sideways in the fall. The horse ran off and left me in a dirt clod field about one mile from where she was stabled.

If a car did not hit her as she crossed the highway, I knew she would be waiting for me in the barn. Slowly I rolled over and stood up, took a few steps, and held my right hand close to my side. I began the mile walk home. Anger made me want to kill my beloved Tennessee Walker horse at that moment. I knew my right breast implant took the brunt of the fall.

Indiana's farmland is my heartland. I left southern Indiana at the age of eighteen when I went to Indiana University, and did not return for sixteen years except for family visits. My childhood had surrounded me with love and horses. At one time, my grandfather had eighteen horses and colts on his farm, and the entire family would gather on Sundays to ride in the Wabash River bottoms near Griffin, Indiana.

My first horse was a palomino named Ribbon. I was eight years old when Grandpa gave me Ribbon, and I had to lead her to a fence gate and climb up the gate to get on her. She was a big gentle Quarter Horse, and I rode her for hours and miles by myself. We only had one accident where she slipped on blacktop and rolled onto my leg. I was bruised but rode her to the barn.

My father bought a companion horse to Ribbon and moved them to a farm closer to my childhood home. I have fond memories of rides near Poseyville and Cynthiana, Indiana, with friends and family. My skill as a rider improved with age, and she died when I was twenty-five years old. After moving to Texas, I rode trail horses and have always been comfortable and confident around horses.

Texas was my home for many years, and I married a co-worker when I was twenty-four years old. I finished my graduate degree in business at the University of Houston, and we moved to San Antonio, Texas, so he could go to dental school. When he graduated from dental school, we moved to Switzerland and lived there almost three years for his work.

During our first year living in Switzerland, a car struck me as I was crossing the road. Standing in the middle of the street, I realized the car could not stop. The car hit me on my thigh and the memory is ingrained. I saw the fear in his eyes as I came up on the hood to meet him. In slow motion: the car, brakes, impact, his eyes, and falling on to the road. I was crossing the road with two sacks of groceries. The milk carton and oats from my sacks exploded onto the road and took the brunt of the impact.

The driver was Italian and I was American, both living in Switzerland as foreigners. I was not using the crosswalk; he had hit a pedestrian. We were both scared, could not communicate, so I did not seek medical help or call the police. I walked away with nothing evidently broken, some numbness in my leg, but no pain. Terrific back pain haunted me for many months afterward. I did not know back pain would follow me for the rest of my life, and the residual weakness would challenge my daily strength. Twenty years later during a chiropractic exam with X-rays, my broken back was discovered.

Skiing was not my strength, but I was in Switzerland, so I skied. I remember one bad tumble while in the French Alps. I negotiated the exit off the lift with an awkward movement and turned to stop. Skiing down one of the slopes, my skis and poles became tangled and I fell, twisting my knee. A gentleman had to put me on his skis to get me down the mountain, and my knee was swollen for several weeks. I never really skied again. I do not get the fun of putting two slick boards on your feet and pointing them down the side of a mountain.

After three years in Switzerland and two years in San Antonio, my marriage of twelve years did not survive. I moved closer to family in Southern Indiana for a job at the local hospital. It was a healing time for me, and I loved being back near farms, cornfields, and horses. My parents lived on a small farm and had a barn, so I started looking for a horse.

After trying out a few, I found Belle, a Tennessee Walker in Kentucky. After being hit by the car in Switzerland, my broken back limited my movement without excruciating pain. I had no pain when I rode Belle because her gait was so smooth. Belle was a spirited, black-coated beauty, and I loved the sense of adventure of riding her and handling her moods. She did not like women, and after my first buck off, I was a bit cautious around her.

We were out for an afternoon ride in a plowed cornfield close to my parent's farm. She was easy to ride and despite the uneven surfaces, I had no pain. Whatever spooked her came as a complete surprise to me, and I was on the ground before I knew what had happened.

I sold the horse.

I thought my multiple illnesses were primarily from treatment effects of chemotherapy, falling skiing, being hit by a car, and being bucked off a horse. It never occurred to me that my implant could leak or rupture. I was never told about any risks.

I feel betrayed by the medical establishment. Five years after my first silicone implant after breast reconstruction in 1987, I was sick constantly. I had no warnings from any physicians, and yet there was something happening to my body.

I decided to write this book, because we do not have an easily available and accepted support group for breast implant illness, except on social media. For women who chose to have breast reconstruction, enhancement or enlargement surgery, we need to discuss the risks and benefits. If few people know you have had implants, it makes it harder to find and discuss the symptoms of breast implant illness. You are not alone. You are not crazy. Trust and listen to your body. It is time to join the community of breast implant illness survivors regardless of where you are in the investigating, receiving an implant, experiencing illnesses, or explanting process.

Chapter 2

First Breast Cancer, First Implant

My breast cancer experience began when I was thirty years old, moving to Switzerland with my husband, working for a hospital and trying to get pregnant. I found a lump in my right breast near the nipple. It was so big and near the surface that my husband saw it from across the room.

We had decided to move to Switzerland when my husband graduated from dental school. He was going to start work first, and I was to join him in a couple months when I finished building a cancer center for my work.

"You need to get that checked out, but I am still leaving for Switzerland in two weeks," he said. His reaction to my potential cancer was scary and hurtful. We had rented out our house and sold our cars. I had resigned my job and was living with a friend.

One month after my husband left for Switzerland, I finally had time for a mammogram. The mammogram revealed a tumor and then the breast biopsy showed malignant cancer. I was scheduled for a mastectomy within a few days. The location of the tumor was very near the nipple and there was no way the general surgeon could effectively remove the tumor and keep the breast shape.

My parents were traveling somewhere in western America. My husband was in Switzerland, and friends were all I had. Mom arrived a couple of days after the diagnosis. My husband came back from Switzerland after my mastectomy and was supportive throughout. Through our friends, we found a new place to live, our car was returned to us after it was sold, and my boss tore up my resignation paper. My husband found a dental research job in a matter of weeks.

The time for treatment would come, but for now, I needed to get back to work. We had to have insurance, and my husband was a new dentist with limited job prospects and no insurance benefits. The decision for chemotherapy, radiation, surgery, and reconstruction were all made within a couple of weeks of surgery. I was also told that I should not plan on ever having children. It was a sad and shocking time of loss.

After the mastectomy, chemotherapy treatment involved Cytoxan, Methotrexate, and 5 FU or CMF for six months. I worked full time and lost some of my hair at the time. I had a tissue expander (another type of implant) placed in the right breast area to help grow new skin so I could get the permanent implant after I received six months of chemotherapy. Every week or two, I visited the plastic surgeon who would insert a needle filled with saline through a port into the tissue expander.

At the end of six months of chemotherapy and one month of recovery, the plastic surgeon inserted a breast implant. My husband and I moved to Switzerland two weeks after my final reconstructive surgery in February 1988. The story of the abrupt end of my marriage in 1992 is detailed in my first book *Deception*.

The plastic surgeon said no skiing this year, but he didn't tell me I couldn't try to ice skate! Which I did! Skiing would have been safer for me because of all my falling on hard ice.

I am a medical technologist and have worked in hospitals and with physicians for most of my career. I have reviewed and kept paper copies of all my medical records from the beginning of cancer in 1987 to explanting in 2016. For the clinically focused readers, I have included detailed medical information.

My first right breast cancer diagnosis was intraductal and infiltrating ductal carcinoma, poorly differentiated Grade III, estrogen and progesterone positive. I had a modified radical mastectomy and the skin, nipple, and all breast tissue with all 27 axillary lymph nodes removed. I had no axillary nodal tumors (the lymph nodes were negative). The tumor was in the upper right quadrant of the breast, 1.5 cm from the nipple. There was evidence of residual breast cancer in the site of the diagnostic biopsy.

The cancer was aggressively growing according to the pathology report. The DNA Flow Cytometry report in 1987 reported that the Diploid DNA Content – S phase showed an increased risk of recurrence based on the node (lymph node) negative patient. Because of being premenopausal and only thirty years old, I took Cytoxan (600 mg/m2) on day one, Methotrexate (40 mg/m2) on days one and eight and 5FU (600 mg/mw on days one and eight through an inserted port in my chest for six months. I tolerated the chemotherapy very well and took one to two days off per month to recover.

The tissue expander was inserted under the pectoralis muscle at the time of the mastectomy and was removed on 1/26/88, seven months after the mastectomy. A Surgitek, 280 cc. adjustable silicone implant was placed in the pocket created by the tissue expander. An additional 50 cc of saline was added for a total volume of 330 cc according to the surgical notes from the plastic and reconstructive surgeon.

In 1988, the FDA issued the polyurethane coated implant warnings. I was never notified or even heard of any risk because of my implant.

Polyurethane-Coated Breast Implants Revisited:
A 30-Year Follow-Up[1]

Dow Corning Corporation manufactured the first silicone gel breast implant in 1962. In the 1970s, a second-generation silicone gel implant was introduced. The new implants were made of silicone, silicone gel, and urethane, and were designed to achieve a natural, safe, and pleasing result that the previous prostheses had failed to achieve [1].

However, in 1988 the Food and Drug Administration (FDA) classified silicone and saline implants as Class III devices, corresponding to the highest level of risk. The FDA required manufacturers of silicone gel-filled breast implants to submit pre-market approval applications with data providing a reasonable assurance of the safety and effectiveness of the implants [2].

In 1991, Surgitek, a manufacturer of polyurethane-coated breast implants, voluntarily withdrew these implants from the market in response to public safety concerns regarding 2,4-toluenediamine (2,4-TDA), a breakdown product of polyurethane [3].

Chapter 3

Pain, No Diagnosis

I have recorded my life through journals since my first breast cancer. Sometimes the journal is a record of what occurred that day, and sometimes it is a concrete record of illnesses I experienced, but never had a diagnosis. I worked in Indiana for a few years until a friend called me to help start a national oncology practice in April 1996. The opportunity was tremendous and the salary was attractive.

After a few years living in Southern Indiana, I had married again. I had sold my horse, and we were both tired of the Indiana winters and ready to move somewhere warmer. I commuted from Indiana to Dallas for six months until we could sell the house and move to Texas in the fall of 1996. I was recording illness after illness in my journals in the spring and summer after I took the new job.

I traveled extensively throughout the United States and loved meeting oncologists and growing this new company. Since I was not even forty years old, I did not share with many people my increasingly poor state of health. My career was taking off, and I had a vice presidency title, travel, and the ability to improve oncology practices throughout the United States. It was an intoxicating time for me to be back in Texas, even though I was asking constantly, "What is wrong with me?" Later that year, I had a physical confirmation that something was very wrong inside my body. There are very explicit clinical issues described in the following journal entries with medical terminology.

Journal

Spring 1996

April 8, 1996

My back was greatly injured years ago and is now mostly recovered. I cannot ever lift heavy things.

April 23, 1996

I am struggling with anal herpes sores. My sciatica is hurting. The pain from my gut is better, but I need to get some medicine.

May 1, 1996

I did not sleep well and woke wide-awake at 1:00 a.m.

Summer 1996

June 1, 1996

Nerves and diarrhea were so bad for 24 hours, I was miserable. We were selling a house and I was exhausted from the closing.

June 4, 1996

My body said "enough" and I was sick with sciatica and back pain.

June 9,1996

Physically I am in pain from feet and hips and uncontrolled bowels at least four times in two weeks. I am beginning to worry and my obsession with bowels leads me to conclude that my body is exhibiting what my brain denies: loss of control, nervousness, sour stomach, and fear. I am praying for healing.

June 14, 1996

My walking has loosened the muscles but increased pain. I feel stress in my lower back with discomfort. The stretching each morning has kept the pain down for several weeks. The severe diarrhea goes on and on. Is it nerves?

June 16, 1996

I am in Hawaii meeting with doctors and there is much to see, but I cannot relax. I have a fever, blisters on my lip, and am tired and sick.

June 24, 1996

Eleven-hour trip with a delayed flight from Chicago to Palm Springs through Los Angeles. It is amazing that the destination controls the traffic coming. It is true in our life as well: our destination determines how and when we get there.

June 27, 1996

Sick again. I started my menstrual bleeding on day twenty and it was very heavy. By the time I get to my hotel in Milwaukee, Wisconsin, I am so weak. I have craved meat two to three times per day, so I wonder if my iron is low?

July 2, 1996

My adrenal glands are swollen on top of my kidneys. They can become inflamed during stress. During a massage, my feet revealed pain in the kidneys, adrenal, and liver. I am taking iron tablets, vitamins, and high doses of vitamin E. Hopefully, I will feel better.

July 11, 1996

Detroit, Michigan, is a city in decline. I had a most embarrassing incident on the tiny plane to Evansville. I had to urinate badly. There were no toilets so my bladder began to cramp. I had to pee. I went to an empty seat in the back and peed in the Barf bag and filled it. I carried it off the plane wrapped in two other bags. Embarrassing.

July 15, 1996

I am at headquarters in Dallas, Texas, with tiredness, tears, and swollen gut from Mexican food and pre-period. I walked, ran, exercised and am in bed by 9:15 p.m. Tired.

July 16, 1996

I cannot read numbers with my left eye with or without glasses. My fingers go numb in my left hand fifteen minutes later. My tongue and throat go numb at fifteen minutes. I cannot hear well. Three hours later after nausea, tests, history, and a peripheral vision test at a neurologist's office, I am diagnosed with complex migraine with neurological involvement. I have to have a brain scan, four vials of blood, weird tests and a $900 bill. Pain and headache. Am I having a stroke?

August 5, 1996

My anti-migraine, anti-depressant works great for me!

August 8, 1996

My stomach is inflamed and I slept until 6:45 a.m. I wake up tired.

August 11, 1996

This weekend is one of recovery after I had an attack Friday night. A headache, great sense of anxiety and doom, and irritability were followed by hot and cold flashes. I have sensitivity to light, lightheadedness, and feeling like I will faint. When I finally slept, it was a sleep of the dead. I am scared because my vision was blurred. God, give me wisdom.

August 22, 1996

Herpes is beginning on my lip. This time it must be stress, as I have had no food or sun problems. I am exhausted.

Fall 1996

September 7, 1996

Twenty-one days with a fever blister and "almost migraine." This has to be hormone related. I feel it coming, take medicine, and go to bed. My vision changes and I cannot see as well. Then the feeling of anxiety comes followed by pressure in my eyes, then a tiny headache and then the blinding headache is followed by light sensitivity.

September 9, 1996

Sick with the flu for the third day with fever, tiredness, and now gut and back pain. What do we do when our bodies fail or rebel? We slow down.

September 16, 1996

Amazing mental exhaustion followed a week in Cincinnati, Ohio. My emotions were up and down. I had fantastic desserts – a dream truffle, salads with blue cheese and walnuts, and pasta with vegetables. (I did not understand the food allergies I had: gluten, dairy, chocolate.)

October 3, 1996

My massage therapist said, "Why do you need the shoulder pain? What is it telling you?" My legs, ribs and back are so sore. Why did I need pain? Pain shows me I am alive and is normal? I did not know I could be without pain? I deserve it? This is starting to affect my mental wellness.

October 5, 1996

I had the beginnings of a migraine and four bowel movements this morning. Is this a release of something or hormonal?

October 8, 1996

My focus is on the pain in my neck, shoulder, and back. I am so tired from jet lag of only one hour traveling to San Diego, California. I have no reserve energy. After I exercised and started my period, the pain disappeared.

October 14. 1996

Tired and out of sorts with fever last night and night sweats. I think I am in early menopause. Do I have HIV? My neck is stiff. What is wrong with me?

October 17, 1996

I had a slight migraine last night. I had an incredible sharp pain above my left eye, then the "feeling" around 5 p.m. and by the time I came home at 7:00 p.m., the migraine was coming on strong. This is the 8th day of my menstrual cycle. What is causing this? Lord, I am scared.

October 25, 1996

We are in Hot Springs, Arkansas, on a four-day vacation. I worked for two hours to get my body to relax. My headache came from a day of no caffeine. My body hurt from the three-hour car ride. I walked, stretched, read, prayed, listened to music, meditated, and slept. How do I maintain balance?

October 29, 1996

I am having trouble taking deep breaths when I returned to work.

Winter 1996

November 4, 1996

Period started on Day 26 and my hormones were wacky. I was crying, screaming, and furious. I want the towel racks put up in the new bathroom and my husband helped me after I screamed at him.

November 10, 1996

I am having trouble focusing my vision right now. Vision is blurry, eye twitches, and head soreness and lights and colors do not seem normal. I have to get into a gynecologist or internist this month for a checkup. I am working 13-hour days and come home beaten up.

November 19, 1996

My neck tension was bad today and has now released with a loud pop. No caffeine as I had three decafs yesterday.

November 22, 1996

I had three wonderful meals in Nashville and ate crème brûlée, tiramisu, salmon with caviar, salads with cheese, cappuccino, pasta salad with shrimp. Then my gut bloats, my knee hurts, and I must change the doctor appointment to later in the week. (Again, I was unaware of the gluten, dairy, and seafood food allergies).

December 1, 1996

My shoulders are giving me great pain and tiredness. My period began with a vengeance, no headache but sensitivity in my left scalp area again. This is my last weekend at home for three weeks.

December 2, 1996

I have pain in my neck from exercise yesterday with constant ringing in my ears. My arm hurts to grip a pen and I have to support it with a pillow to write. I cannot carry anything anymore. I am awake at 1:20 after two hours of tossing and turning. The pain in my head goes to my neck to my shoulders.

and my arms. My anger is rolling down my face in painful sobs. As I cry, the pain subsides in my arms as I release my growing distress.

December 3, 1996

Massage taught me another lesson: my body will scream for the pain I cannot allow myself to feel. I fell on my right armpit crossing those hanging bars at the gym. My left side was screaming in pain.

When the massage therapist was working the shoulders, she found **"a huge knot around my right implant."** She stopped and said, "Doesn't that hurt?" I felt nothing but the referred pain in my neck and left shoulder. Weird.

I traveled to California, Missouri, and Indiana the next week for business and personal visits before the holidays.

December 25, 1996

I am still battling flu with severe diarrhea and took a two-hour nap. My stomach is so tender from the abdominal cramps, residual migraine, and herpes sore on my tongue and vagina. It was not a healthy holiday.

December 29, 1996

My mammogram was all right, but they did an ultrasound to look at some nodules. They look fine. I was calm and prayed while they checked me for cancer.

The pain and illness journey continued throughout 1997 while I was working, traveling, and trying to cope with increasing symptoms and illnesses. Cancer re-enters my life within eighteen months, but I kept up the grueling schedule of travel to oncologist's offices across the nation.

Journal

Winter 1997

January 1, 1997

I have a small headache and eye twitch today from a migraine yesterday. This is the third one in ten days plus flu, plus period, and a mammogram. I need to lose ten pounds.

January 6, 1997

I am saddened by my first signs of aging at thirty-nine with stiffness in joints, decreasing eyesight and tiredness even with eight hours of sleep.

January 7, 1997

My gynecologist called and said my blood work was normal, except my blood sugar was high. Am I a diabetic at almost forty? Should I go on Tamoxifen as I am already spending so much on medicine?

January 18, 1997

I had a headache on day 23 of my period. I drank some Asti Spumante last night and am tight, irritable, quiet and in pain. I have a little anal sore starting again.

January 22, 1997

A migraine hit last night so I took one pill in the evening. My neck was so tight and I almost had two wrecks getting to work and coming home. My stress was a nine out of ten. I am so angry.

January 28, 1997

Another migraine knocked me out last night in San Diego. The basis seems to be tension especially in my neck. I want a massage badly. I slept ten hours and took another pill but cannot function well. Am I living the life I want? What do I want more of? Quality time, not so rushed. What do I want less of? Stress.

January 30, 1997

Lord, I am weary. I have work to do, and no energy. God, help me pace myself, keep a good perspective and be Christ-like.

February 1, 1997

My body is tired from the massage yesterday. My neck was tight and feels beaten up today.

February 4, 1997

I am in Houston and Harlingen, Texas, this week and am sick with a cold and sore throat. My immune system collapsed after the massage. I spent all day on the couch and went to bed at 5:30 p.m. The sore throat is better and the congestion has eased. I am sick more than I would like.

February 5, 1997

My throat still hurts badly, but my ears are not hurting after the medicine. I hope to slowly recover this week. I am tired of being sick and fighting illness daily or at least weekly.

February 12, 1997

I am finally recovered after ten days of cold, sore throat, fever and diarrhea. I was in Harlingen, Houston, and Dallas, Texas; St. Louis, Columbia, Jefferson City, and St. Charles, Missouri last week.

February 19, 1997

My vision is blurring and changing with the "under the surface" headache. My vision must be checked for continuing weakness and change. I may need glasses constantly soon. I spent the day in Austin, Round Rock, and Waco, Texas.

February 23, 1997

I am trying to shake this weak voice and heaviness in my chest. According to casual oncologist conversations, I should go on Tamoxifen. **I read an article in *Newsweek* about the unique immune disease for silicone implants.**

February 26, 1997

Tired again! The tickle in my throat goes on forever. I work out every day for 30-45 minutes with weights and aerobics.

February 28, 1997

I am in Spokane, Washington, after driving to Coeur d'Alene, Idaho, to visit an oncology center. I felt so bad when I arrived yesterday. After sleeping nine hours, I went to a minor emergency center and got antibiotics. My temperature was down finally after antibiotics.

Spring 1997

March 10, 1997

I have herpes on my lip and anus again, so I took medicine and hope to halt it getting worse. San Diego again with a late flight and very stressed with all the meetings.

March 19, 1997

Forty years old birthday and ten years post cancer. I went to get my Clinique makeup and the girl said, "Clinique is focused on younger skin." Thanks, I needed that today.

March 24, 1997

I am tired of being sick all the time! I had an allergic swelling reaction in my knee and soreness throughout my body. Weight is 138 pounds, and I cannot lose weight. Headaches are from what? Irritability constantly, and if I drink alcohol, I pay for it. If I take antibiotics, I get infected from an allergic reaction.

March 31, 1997

I slept three hours and was exhausted with a sore throat.

April 2, 1997

As predicted, I crashed in Waco, Texas. Sore throat, fever, fever sores inside my mouth. I ate bread with olive oil, pasta with crispy crawfish (I did not know I was allergic to shellfish and sensitive to gluten).

April 9, 1997

San Diego, Poway, and Mission Valley, California. I have made it two months without a severe headache. Exercise, massage, no wine, and very limited caffeine. I am taking Vitamin B6 and Vitamin C in high amounts. Lord, I am tired today.

April 13, 1997

I had a massage and she unblocked some channels. I must stop focusing my body's attention on "weak" parts and keep all parts in balance. My right arm and shoulder were in great pain, and I was ignoring it because I do not feel pain anymore. I told my massage therapist, "This right side is dead." Harmful words. I ran in a 5K as a breast cancer survivor. Taking Vitamin C 1500-2500 mg per day, Vitamin E for reduction in headaches and protein three times a week, and I have energy again. Work is very stressful and I cried in my office after being verbally attacked by a co-worker.

April 18, 1997

I had a semi-bad accident in California with the two doctors from La Jolla. Of course, I injured my neck and back as I was driving. I had a premonition that they should drive, but ignored it. There were parked cars on the street and have no idea where the other driver came from. I had to go to the police station, and then drive the car to Hertz to get another rental. My neck and back were stiff within the hour, so later I used ice, then hot bath, took a muscle relaxer to help it heal.

I flew to St. Louis, Missouri, followed by 3.5 hours drive to Kirksville, then a two-hour drive to Columbia, Missouri, after this accident. I drove to Lake of the Ozarks, Missouri, to meet with doctors, back to Columbia and 2-hour drive to St Louis. Too much!

April 29, 1997

Spokane, Washington, visits through Salt Lake City, Utah. Now I need a crown on my sore tooth. This is an unexpected health expense. I know it will be positive to remove the mercury fillings and replace them with a composite crown. I have had the filling for 25 years.

May 5, 1997

I weigh 142 pounds, up another 4 pounds, headache, premenstrual, and tired. I cannot lose weight. God, help those in my way today.

May 10, 1997

Massage today and tremendous pain from the accident. With the tooth and the wreck, there is built-up body pain that makes me mean!

May 15, 1997

I visited family and Rocky Mountain National Park for a couple days before an oncology conference in Denver. I walked through a herd of elk after hiking 7.5 miles of trails.

May 21, 1997

We stood at the booth at the oncology conference from 8 a.m. until 12:00 p.m. for three straight days. I am tired.

May 30, 1997

My feet hurt badly and itch in the middle. I itch on my arms, back, dry skin and constant scratching. It must be nerves. The sense I have is there is always something wrong with my body. I am seven days from my period and have not taken any medicine for one week. I take my vitamins and homeopathy medicine to try to get through one month without a headache. Why am I a "space cadet?"

Summer 1997

June 10, 1997

Sores on my buttocks, right leg pain, and a cold for three days. I exercised and went back to bed. Obviously, I am not doing well. It is so scary to deal with this cyclical sex thing. Do I have a sexually transmitted disease? I have decided to not take Tamoxifen, go off my headache medicine, and watch carefully my alcohol, salt, and food intake.

I did a calendar check and have had seven colds, sore throat, lip/mouth sores, four migraines, tooth problem, accident/wreck and foot hurting from nerves, and four times with anal sore in six months. Every two weeks, something is wrong as I am barely functioning. Now, what do I do about it? My exhaustion is from my body battling all of this. If I were healthy, how much living could I do? I must share this with a medical person. It is not normal to be having immune system problems every two weeks.

June 16, 1997

I have fought severe joint pain and allergic sores for a few days and am scared of this illness or what it means. Work pressures leave me trapped and resentful. My neck is tight and it is time for a massage.

July 1, 1997

I slept eight hours. My throat is swollen each morning and my right knee hurts. My body is failing me in many ways.

July 7, 1997

I have lived ten years after my breast cancer diagnosis. Is it fun to be alive at 40? Where do I go now? What would I do if I do not have to constantly recover? I will stay in Dallas for ten days and reflect on this question.

July 9, 1997

Sick again with fever and cold sore on mouth. My nose is runny and I am tired. It is day 12 of menstrual cycle and my whole lip is infected and I had a headache when I awoke. Something is very wrong. I feel as if I am in a precarious balance and anything pushes me over the edge to illness. The doctor tomorrow at my appointment will examine the sore on the anal area. The doctor gave me medicine for herpes to take daily.

July 14, 1997

Illness is apparent with two one-hour naps, but at least I did not fall in bed exhausted. My nose and cheeks are inflamed, I have fear of losing my eyesight, and my ears burn inside. It does look like herpes, but only opportunistically or when my immune system is weak. I think it was a bee sting on my upper lip. The bumps and itching on my face make me think of the sting. It is just like the drug allergy. When will this get better?

July 22, 1997

I have napped twice today and am very tired and sick to my stomach with cramps. Even my liver feels sore and I have stomach cramps. A half-day of sick time would be good, but I cannot. I am embarking on rehabilitation, healing, and a low, slow climb-out of the last ten years. My bowel movement is very loose. I am taking medicine while I heal. Of course, I feel worse when "detoxing" my body.

August 1, 1997

I will be gone most of this month traveling and preparing for changes at work. I must make appointments for doctor, massage, and a nutritionist.

August 9, 1997

I had a massage at the Seattle, Washington, airport after a trip to Eugene, Oregon, on the way to San Diego, California. I am always rushing, but I cannot "close" the doctor deals.

August 19, 1997

I fell twice yesterday; once on an escalator in Mall of America and once in my hotel room in St. Paul, Minnesota.

August 23, 1997

The deadline is set for October 1, 1997. If no deal is closed, I am fired. Pain of possible change again. My journey is almost over here. My pride must be shattered again. God has a window for me if this door closes.

August 30, 1997

Lincoln, New Mexico, is the home of Billy the Kid, and we are staying at the Casa de Patron. I have had a migraine today, as I did not sleep well in El Paso, Texas, last night. I was fighting with stomach cramps and tight neck all day long. This is my third "near episode" this week. The work stress is greater than I realize. I know my shoulders are tight constantly. We slept well on this vacation, but no sexual desire.

Fall 1997

September 10, 1997

I have a reprieve of six months to close hospital deals, if none are closed with these doctors, I will be fired. My roller coaster of emotions is ongoing. My hands are going numb all the time and my sleep is interrupted in two-hour segments. I have to exercise or I am lost.

September 12-September 27, 1997

When I was on vacation for two weeks in Europe, I have no problems with my health. I assume the issues are work and stress.

October 3, 1997

Working and commuting takes twelve hours per day. I sleep eight hours. My exercise and grooming are two hours a day. Not much time off and this cannot go on forever.

October 8, 1997

I am in a fog. I went to the doctor with such an earache and fever yesterday. Then my friend who was my boss was fired. I moved here to this company to work with her. What a day!

October 24, 1997

Massage last week helped with the neck pain, but I cried the following morning. I took ten minutes and listened to music yesterday, which was my first relaxation in three weeks.

Winter 1997

November 2, 1997

Ear herpes, period, insomnia, gas, overwhelming pain, and I have to go to work tomorrow and travel all week.

November 13, 1997

No period yet and I am 10 days late. Weird.

December 22

Migraine again with head pain and vision affected. Two migraines in two weeks and beginning of another sore are tough. Seems like carbohydrate withdrawal. Should I continue to push myself?

December 31, 1997

The green and yellow ooze of tingling started in my arm, waking me once more to numbness. As I slowly turned in bed, the numbness turned into searing icicles. Pain became my companion within seconds.

Sometimes the massage is healing for a moment. When it gets too bad, there is medicine. But I hoard the medicine like I hide my chocolate. I only take half, never whole pills. I am trying to win a badge of courage and the will of tolerance.

Walking, talking, sex, and going to the bathroom are all taken for granted until the companion of pain overrides the ease in me. First the shoulder pain, then the stomach pain migrates to the breast surgery scar moving to the knee through the back, up the neck, then into the head exploding in sores in the mouth and anus. All contribute a part to my constant companion of quiet pain. It is totally private in this world. No one understands the silence, the drawn eyes, and the energy-draining companion of pain.

Unless you experience it, you believe you can "will it away" or just push it deep within your soul. It is like a predatory animal, quietly stalking you in circles of icicles and slowly sneaks up on you. Then wham, you are stopped as if dead in your stillness.

I must kick in the controlled breathing. I must concentrate completely on putting the pain monster back in its cage. Hoping there will be at least a level of winning. Not settling for odds of survival, slamming the door on the monster, and I am holding the key in my sweaty and terrified hands.

February 1, 1998

The women I thought about today were the "suffering sisters." It was not a club anyone wanted to belong to or be in today. Cancer. Cancer has a requirement with tragedy as the main character. It will forever shape your life with the firmness of ceramics molded on a wheel and dried. My life had been over twice, so I developed strong opinions about everything. I was a miracle of survival and believed in the impossible. God is merciful and strengthens me like gold and diamonds. He is creating, sharpening, shaping, honing, and cutting, and making me into His masterpiece.

February 16, 1998

Scary and fear-filled dream starts my morning. I do not want to go to work. I pursue the emptiness of my dream of being fulfilled at work. When the uselessness of commerce becomes obvious, at what point do I give up? I need to rest for six months in the mountains. Fear is my ugly companion now.

February 18, 1998

I am sad today. There is death all around my periphery. Cremation is cheap and the burial of an urn is less than I thought. My grandfather is in the hospital and is saying his good-byes. He told me, "I love you, too." First time in forty years I heard that from him.

My pain tolerance is very high, both emotional and physical. I received seven shots of anesthesia yesterday to knock me out of this pain. I may be allergic slightly, but I came home and slept. Death permeates the week.

February 19, 1998

How do I "lie low" and coast at work? I need to rest from all the travel. How much time must pass as I wait to be fired? I am sure dead people were not talking about work at their death. They thought of family, friends, and relationships, but not work. I have been watching the skaters on the Olympics. Their eyes and face light up when they are successful and doing exactly what they want. How long since I felt that way? We put our house up for sale to get ready for change. I will not "should" myself about the past. There is no clear path forward, I only know change is on the horizon.

February 24, 1998

I could not get up today with a residual migraine from only five hours sleep. Rollerblades? Why haven't I bought them? It is like my bike, I am too busy to get the bike down and use it. My coping mechanism is weakened. Two days later, my neck is tight and my stomach hurts! Tension and I do not want to be at work and cannot wait to leave. Seems like too much of an effort today to keep writing. I will write affirmations today.

February 25, 1998

It was a good day until I missed my flight. I hauled my crap into the bathroom, changed clothes, bought a big latte and bugged the flight attendant for a seat. Has this been only one day? Before noon, I was exercising, been sick, traveled, packed, ate lunch, been on a treadmill for a cardiology exam, and took a nap. I took a standby. No wonder travel is exhausting.

February 26, 1998

I have concern for my mental health, but there is also genuine fear. My brain is unclear as in a fog. How do you truly keep going in exhaustion? First, I use stimulants. Second, I take naps and rest. Third, I go slower. The exhaustion causes me to not use my brain. It is good to remember the opportunities for silence are greater than the opportunities for constant discussion. In reality, there are a few internal truths, but most thoughts are individual perceptions of reality.

February 27, 1998

My travel experiences are getting crowded with more people, more roll-on suitcases, and less space. The way home is spent lifting, hauling, pushing, and pulling the luggage. The strain on my upper body is excruciating. I have started lifting weights regularly to forestall damage, and it helps.

It is lonely to be the only female in the "den" of lions or thieves. That is why "bitch" is associated with strength. It is confusing for all men and women. Saying no to the men and know they will still respect me is a science and an art. Perhaps a leave of absence is all I truly need? It takes courage to walk away from these financial opportunities.

Tiredness shows itself to me in my inability to recover quickly. Exhaustion, breakdown of systems, so much stress and pressure to make money and achieve.

Spring 1998

March 2, 1998

Six months of having an ax over my head at work. Does it do any good to threaten people to make them succeed? If I do not sell, I am a failure. If I sell into this mess, I am a failure to my client. I will take the former. The need to escape and rest is real. Lord, you will not give me more than I can bear. Keep me safe. I do not want to make another mistake. It has been a hard life with much weariness.

March 7, 1998

I slept until 6:40 a.m. and feel better today. My chest and head are still thick, but fever peaked last night. If I have only six months to live or eighteen months, what would I do? Meeting the needs of my inner health with no outward focus is like being on a seesaw dangerously out of balance. When I leave and where I go to is not in my hands, but in God's hands. My messed-up workaholic ventures coupled with a sense of urgency delight me when I receive recognition. Thinking that money provides me protection is certainly the fallacy of commerce.

March 9, 1998

What will I do today? I am quiet with the pain and shame of herpes. It starts with a quiet burning, tenderness and tingling follows. My hot flash coincides with the heat inside and out. Two out of three nights I have a cold, fever, or am pre-menopausal. Everyone is leaving this place. They have either resigned or been fired.

Perhaps God wants us to float and settle where He wants us to be, not where He puts me. I keep moving. The overwhelming need to change every two years does not create an environment for more than cursory relationships. I cry over things of deep meaning. Am I taking time off through illness?

March 14, 1998

My sadness over all the people leaving and loss translated into my body. I told myself, "Shut up, why can't you keep your mouth shut?" and I promptly lost my voice for two days. I stayed at home with illness for two days and felt crummy another two days. An illness gave me the badly needed rest I craved.

The team disintegrates. Change is coming quickly. I am writing stories of my dreams and experiences. I need counseling. Does God have to take away all the things I have achieved in order to get me to do what He wants me to do?

March 25, 1998

Children are lured to their deaths by a fake fire drill. I awoke to a murderous dream and it is not a great start to the day so I napped for a while. What is this need to "keep going" all about today? I was gone for eleven days and slept in eight different beds in ten days. My weariness is more of a battle of the heart, soul, and emotions. Knowing my limitations and pushing past that point makes me know how strong my mind is over my weakened body.

After getting up and dressed, the weariness sets in. I want to go back to bed. How can I go on at this pace? Weariness, and I fear some depression and anger are surfacing. Burn out.

March 30, 1998

We sold our house and will move out two years after moving into our house. We have no jobs and we will rest for a few weeks. Why did I resign? I want my life back and this is no life. I visualize my health as one year with no herpes or viral infection.

April 7, 1998

Rest will decrease illness. The herpes attack this time is so painful. The pain down my leg to my knee is so severe. I spent time on foot massage in the evening to release muscles. Pain was relieved with aspirin and stretching. My lymph nodes are swollen in the groin. I have cramps and swollen ovaries and a migraine and am miserable.

April 16, 1998

I am finished, done, spent, and exhausted. I do not sleep normally; I slumber in the sleep of death. Anywhere, anyhow, I doze. My tiredness is a boring subject. I am rough and angry with people on the phone and in person. I am not kind. I sat on my couch and covered up in the wedding quilt of 17 years ago and cried. Sad, alone, and exhausted. I take muscle relaxers or alcoholic drinks to sleep, and then wake up at the end not rested.

April 19, 1998

I slept for eleven hours and have no energy for anything. My neck is so tense as I lay in the sun with a residual headache. I want to do nothing. There is no interest or ability to have sex. April seems to be the month for my depressions and crashing. It seems to be a pattern: hard work, unsettled environment, pain, distrust, alone, and no one to help. I promised to work six more months and I did it. I always do what I have to in order to be successful, survive, and achieve.

April 27, 1998

I do not have the energy to reach out to my friends or my husband. I am mean, and he is tired and I do not care. This marriage suffers an enormous strain with a loss of intimacy tantamount to living as roommates. My eye begins its self-flickering and everything blurs in the light.

I sleep and sleep the sleep of the emotionally sick, but I must hide it for fear of being wrongly judged. No one would understand my blues, sadness, and no facial affect. I am burned out and know the meaning of illness once again. People ask me how I do it all, and now I can say, "I can't." Physically and mentally it is so hard to keep going at this pace. I can't. I am resigning from this job.

May 5, 1998

Herpes and ear infection again. PMS and migraine. If there is to be recovery, it starts with rest and with God. I am bouncing from fear to negative emotions to joy to anxiety in thirty minutes. "Dark times of the soul." Moving through the weeks in a fog of remembrance and fatigue. Finished negotiating stock options, vacation, and severance package. In three weeks, I am out.

May 17, 1998

I have one big trip to an oncologist convention in Los Angeles before I am finished at work. I am feeling lost and overwhelmed. The exhaustion once again sets in, as it is impossible to pace myself. Up at 5:30 a.m. California time. Traveling 10,000 miles per month seems excessive to most people.

I saw many of the oncologists I knew from San Antonio. We ate at a great restaurant in Hollywood. My feet hurt and I have had no exercise, only standing for hours. I cannot seem to remember names well and the tiredness is creeping back. I went to the Getty Museum and I am staying at the Westin Bonaventure. The amount of experiences and stimuli I have experienced through this job is amazing. All the opportunities, potentials, travel, and excitement wore me down. It has been a privilege.

My job ended at the end of May 1998. I resigned to one of the doctor managers on a trip to Minneapolis. The extensive travel and company difficulties had left me exhausted. It was a tiredness that was only felt by cancer survivors. I knew I was on a downward spiral into cancer again. When I spoke to one of my co-workers at that time, they had no idea how sick I was. She said, "Working for those doctors, we could not show any sign of weakness."

We did not know where we were going to live and picked three cities to evaluate in the West. Tulsa, Oklahoma; Victoria, Texas; and Colorado Springs, Colorado, were on the top of our potential destinations, and we planned trips to stay in each of them for a week. We wanted smaller cities, near military bases with good weather and lots of sunshine. I never want to live where there are helicopters reporting on traffic. We began to prepare everything for storage until we decide where to live and find employment.

The symptoms of breast implant illness are all there, and I have only four months before cancer is diagnosed again.

Chapter 4

Second Breast Cancer

I n the summer of 1998, we sold our house, traveled to find a new home, and were unemployed. We experienced a kind of homelessness and spent time crashing with friends we knew around the country.

I made a decision in July that I would have my implant removed in the fall when we were settled. Why is that in my journal? Chronic illness had plagued me for a few years, and there was something in my intuition that said, "get the implant out of your body."

Journal

Summer 1998

June 30, 1998

I have depressing weight gain and am premenstrual. I am not soliciting work, and opportunities are coming to me. It makes me nauseous thinking about working again. I know I will be all right and going forward will be in God's plan. I look forward to great health from good food and healthy vitamins.

July 2, 1998

A potential migraine is looming and I am fighting it with medicine. My health is so much better.

July 5, 1998

I am awakened with bad herpes and pain in my hip and leg last night. My anxiety is high when I think about work again. The pain lasted two hours and I went to sleep at 3 a.m. I am on Day 31 of my cycle and no period.

July 7, 1998

Eleven years ago today my life was changed with the words, "Debi, I am sorry you have cancer." I was 30 years old and alone with friends. I asked for 25 more years from God and eleven have already passed. My July 7 verse from the Bible is Ephesians 3:20.

July 9, 1998

I am lying on the floor after painful bleeding and passing a huge clot after gardening this morning. Sleep is elusive with no more than three hours at a time for two nights. My husband and I are fighting horribly and my anger explodes.

July 10, 1998

I have decided to remove my implant this fall. I am tired of allergic reactions to Chinese food, ant bites, and knees are swollen. I have experienced burns and cuts to my skin.

July 16, 1998

Incredible view of purple and blue mountains capped with pink against the blue and black storm sky in Taos, New Mexico. I am exhausted from the move.

July 17, 1998

My pain level is pretty high today for some reason. Driving three hundred miles doesn't help. Rolling burnt prairie to the majesty of the mountains that are covered with clouds and scrub brush. The fierceness of the blue sky is a place of rest as it turns your head to the heat. We now go to Colorado for ten days. Perhaps I will recover some from this weariness. My physical pain is very real.

July 18, 1998

Colorado Springs at rush hour is easy but a bit hectic. Old Colorado City and the Garden of the Gods are out my front door. This town is high on my list of relocation possibilities.

July 21, 1998

I was very sick with diarrhea on the "Million Dollar Highway" on our way to Durango and Silverton, Colorado, for a train trip. It was a gorgeous drive across the mountains.

We spent a week at the XF Ranch above the Black Canyon of Gunnison, Colorado. Horseback riding in mountain meadows, viewing stands of huge aspen, sheer shale rock fall, streams, and going up and down mountains. The rocking of the horse lulled me with a sense of peace.

The sounds stayed in my memories. Horse hoofs crossing shale and water run-offs, which stretch far up and down the mountains. We could hear the creek's running water and the gentle lapping of the lake water. The bear I saw was big enough to see across a mountain valley as it crossed the snowpack. The bear stopped and stared at us while we were watching it. I had a dream and was so sad as I was totally ignored as if I did not exist. I am too weak to fight.

July 27, 1998

I am full of energy and positive enthusiasm back home in Cynthiana, Indiana, near Evansville. I hope to help Mom through her surgery recovery. My body felt the car ride from Colorado to Indiana, as it is always difficult for me to ride long distances in a car. My parents are full of energy, and I seem to have nothing to offer to them.

I had tears and some emotion comes from the tiredness, and I had a realization of the preciousness of life. Hold life tightly, but squeeze it lightly. Time goes quickly and all we are left with is our connected humanity keeping us sane in a crazy world.

Journal

Summer 1998

August 1, 1998

I am in my hometown and I am in hiding. Rest, blessed rest. My period started on Day 21, and I was crazy, poisoned by the estrogen. I cried, had suicidal thoughts, and felt bad with diarrhea and cramping. A migraine followed the next day and mom asked, "Are you pregnant?"

I have not felt good for two days and cannot get anything done. Exhaustion.

August 6, 1998

I have slept the sleep of death for days. My dreams are vivid, but I was awake through a restless pain-filled night. I was mowing for my parents and the riding lawn mower jerked me enough to cause my neck and back to "go out." My back does not allow much trauma and it is good to know this. I sleep 8–9 hours and then nap every day. My neck felt unstable and Mom rubbed it twice to help the pain.

August 16, 1998

Pain, in all its glory, moves across every area of my back. It is slowly moving from one side to the other. I hurt my back on a waterslide and have a right lower back spasm with pain on any movement. Four muscle relaxers and bed rest yesterday. Mom rubbed my back twice and I slept on ice. Now it is stiff again. I cannot take this pain much longer.

I had so hoped my health would drastically improve without the stress of work. So, I will try to move forward even with this pain. All the moving, car trips, hiking, lawn mowing proved to be too much, and the burdens show through my back pain.

This is like living with a disability. I must see why this right side of my body is so messed up. **Take out the implant.** I have pain in my ovaries, pimples, right knee and right hip pops when I walk. I always have to move and exercise or I become unable to move.

Lord, teach me the quiet lessons of rest and focus on you alone.

The radiologist thinks there is a rupture of the silicone implant. Finally, a possible reason for being so sick for so long.

August 19, 1998

Very little sleep, maybe five hours, hot, itching, pain, and fever – basic herpes attack. I am so tired of being sick. Thank you, Lord for this time of sharing with my mom, rest and laughter. Being with family is a blessing.

My second breast cancer was diagnosed in September 1998, eleven years after the first breast cancer. I found new cancer, a lump on the left breast that summer, and I hoped it was not a re-occurrence. Surgery and reconstruction were scheduled in Dallas, Texas, and I worked with a breast oncologist and plastic surgeon to remove the right silicone implant and have it replaced with a saline implant at the same time as the lumpectomy. I had no idea the silicone implant had actually ruptured. Life changed drastically for me again.

How long was I sick before the second breast cancer? Four years. Four years since I was bucked off a horse and landed on my right silicone implant.

Journal

Fall 1998

September 8, 1998

I have a lump in my left breast but am not saying anything to my parents. We have not worked for three months, so after our trip to Washington, DC for Dad's 60th birthday, we must return to packing and finishing projects. **I want to remove my implant this fall.** We are moving to Colorado Springs, Colorado, and are taking our time driving from Indiana through Kansas to the "first view" of the Rockies.

September 16, 1998

My dream takes place at the end of a long day, and I am alone at a park. The swimming pool is empty. I have swum there and was visibly topless with one implant and one breast. The feeling was that I was at the end, the completion of the journey. I am finally going home to rest from the park with unbelievable tiredness and weariness.

Now, another mammogram to look at this little bump. My life could change instantly and I want to talk with my friends. The similarities to eleven years ago are so great: I can walk, but not run five miles, no permanent home, living with others, preparing to pick up our things from Dallas, and move to the mountains with my husband's job. It is all so similar to eleven years ago after the first cancer.

September 19, 1998

I have the diagnosis of breast cancer again eleven years later. I knew it from the second set of pictures, from the shiny dots of calcification on the screen with blown-up pictures and from the dark mass on the ultrasound. One large area is about 1.5 cm like my first cancer tumor but located in the upper outer quadrant of the left breast. It was palpable to the doctor.

This is only six months to the day since my last Pap smear and breast examination, and nothing was there at that time.

I decided I wanted to be treated in Texas where I knew the cancer care was excellent. The radiologist suggested a needle biopsy to "confirm" cancer. Shoot. Not now. Not again.

I fell at my friend's house and have a big bruise on my hip and a sore right shoulder. I am sore on my left breast and tired of sleeping on my back. Ten days of rest and healing when I felt happy and whole. I have appointments with Dr. A, breast surgeon and with Dr. P, the plastic surgeon, on Monday.

God, what does this all mean? How much of my life must still be surrendered to God's sovereignty? It will be the hardest thing I do. "That is enough. I cannot go on in my own power. You have to help me keep going, Lord." My sobbing begins to release the pain.

My journal scripture that day was Psalms 147:4 (NASB), "He counts the number of the stars; He gives names to all of them."

My husband asked me to never give up. I told him I could not promise that, not yet, but to keep asking.

These eleven years have been so valuable to me: people, places, and things to see and do. The dearness of life each day is clear to me. Satan is a liar and prayer is holding back my fear of death. I know shock and tears will come in waves next week.

September 20, 1998

Awoke with a migraine with a gray filter. My left shoulder hurts and it scares me. Bone cancer already? I have numbness in my hand and fingers and a swollen breast from the procedure. Alive. At church, I was crying through the music. My ear has been ringing, and I have not yet started treatments.

Lord, I want to be healed. At least make me fun and functional. I promise to do for others, and increase my own courage to live.

My husband's tears are a constant reminder of his private pain. He shows a specter of unbelievable sadness. I wake him every night to talk, laugh, love, and cry. We go to sleep cuddled in mutual comfort.

Lord, let the shield cut off blood to the tumor and put a stop to peripheral and stray cells. Let the net be pulled over it and stop the arm pain.

September 21, 1998

I have soreness and tenderness in my left foot and brown in the "reflexology" area of the breast. Life goes on at our friend's house where we are staying near Dallas. Nausea is a constant companion, and I think my mind and body are finally fighting. It is a long journey, so hang on for the ride.

I saw the plastic surgeon to discuss having the implant removed from the right breast and replaced with a new saline implant at the same time as my cancer surgery. Surgery will probably be a lumpectomy.

September 22, 1998

I called the research physician today, who I knew from my time at my oncology center job to ask three things: Would she consult with me? Yes. Is two weeks all right to wait for surgery? Yes. Is my breast surgeon worth waiting for to see? Yes. She asked, "Would I take an experimental drug known to shrink tumors in metastatic patients?" They were running a small Phase II trial test on 35 patients before breast surgery, if they would stay on the medicine ten days. It is not FDA approved yet.

Sign me up! I cannot stand to do nothing to fight cancer. I received the drug that day after signing eight pages of consent forms.

September 25, 1998

The Internet shows no survival difference between a lumpectomy plus radiation and a simple mastectomy. Re-occurrence is high (30-40%) with positive lymph nodes. Damn depressing to have this disease again.

God, what am I to teach others: courage, dependency, acceptance, and to live every day fully? How do I deal with this need for attention? I know life goes on, but I want their company not prayers. What is my body's desire to keep dying? Pain and illness make me want to quit living.

The breast surgeon was interested to operate after someone has taken the experimental drug and see what effects it had on the tumor. Great news.

The research doctor said, "We cure 1.5 cm tumors all the time." The tumor was big enough to be felt, and I am glad I only waited a few months.

We are ready to have our own space, not to live in someone else's house. We have ten days when our host is gone at this house. Lord, thank You for unbelievable timing.

"My life closed twice before its close"
Emily Dickinson

My life closed twice before its close—
It yet remains to see
If immortality unveils
A third event for me,
So huge, so hopeless to conceive
As these that twice befell.
Parting is all we know of heaven
And all we need of hell.

September 24, 1998

Naps followed a stress-filled and exhausting morning. The liver and lymph node tests were completed, and I met with the surgeon. She really wants me to do lumpectomy with radiation. Good reasons are the location of the tumor, cure rate, and good chemotherapy drugs.

I explained the emotion, not the science, was my reluctance. Keeping my breast is not important. Living is what I want. I want no regrets and no "I wish I would have…" I also have the issue of the **removal of the implant. The radiologist thinks there is an encapsulated rupture of the implant.**

September 27, 1998

It itches. The whole area itches including under my arm. Is the experimental treatment killing the tumor? There are palpable changes. The drug made me a little sick today. I rest after I take the drug. I do not know what I did to deserve this. But of course, we did nothing to deserve this second cancer at 41 years of age.

Where do I go with this anger? I am mad at God. Why do I have to struggle? Why must I begin to once again think about my death? I am so angry that I am sick with cancer again.

I am so angry that I have to ask for help again.

I am so angry that my body has to heal.

I am so angry that I must perform and keep going, even if I want to give up.

I am so angry that I am homeless, without insurance, and have no job and no insurance benefits. Yes, I have COBRA that I am paying so I am covered for eighteen months.

I am so angry that I have not taken better care of myself. I knew I needed to stop the work pace.

Get a grip on your mind and thoughts.

I am so happy I had eleven years without cancer. It is so much better diagnostically and medically than my previous cancer. I am so glad that I rested this summer and am lucky to be surrounded by love and still be alive. I am pleased I knew who to go to for medical help in Dallas and am surrounded by the hospitality of friends. I will learn about giving it all to God again, and am God's child. That is enough for me.

I am a medical technologist and often moved, so I kept paper copies of all my medical records. I have included my clinical notes on the second breast cancer, left side diagnosed September 19, 1998. It starts with a negative mammogram I had seven months before this cancer was diagnosed.

Diagnostic Mammogram – March 4, 1998, (only seven months before cancer)

Impression: No change from 1996

1. Dense nodular breast parenchyma without interval change from the prior study in December 1996.
2. A left mammogram in one year is recommended.

Sonographic Needle Biopsy Texas Women's Imaging – September 19, 1998

1. 1.5 cm irregular solid mass associated with calcification located at the 2 o'clock position, 7 cm from the nipple. The histologic findings are malignant.
2. The hyalinized stroma is infiltrated by nests and sheets of malignant cells with enlarged hyperchromatic nuclei, which vary considerably in size and shape.

Whole Body Bone scan - negative

Echocardiogram - normal

Medical City Dallas - Ambulatory Surgical Report 10/98
Diagnosis:
1. Stage III, 1.8 cm, high grade infiltrating duct carcinoma of the left breast diagnosed 9/98. Direct extension into an intramammary node, and 1 of 20 axillary nodes. Her-2-Neu negative. Estrogen receptor negative and progesterone receptor positive.
2. **Possible altered immune status due to silicone breast implants.**
3. Preoperative DFMO (experimental chemotherapy) 10 days prior to left breast lumpectomy. In 10/98 her silicone implant was removed and a saline implant placed in the right breast.
4. Severe toxicity with Cytoxan and Adriamycin noted on 11/3/98.

Surgical Pathology Consultation
Medical City Dallas 10/5/1998

Biologic implant capsule from right breast: Sclerosis; scattered clusters of vacuolated macrophages are present; no neoplastic changes are identified. Silicone implant from right breast – grossly intact silicone capsule.

Specimen J is designated right breast capsule and is a collapsed membranous segment of tissue measuring up to 22 cm in maximum dimension and 0.3-0.4 cm in thickness. The inner surface is smooth and free of calcifications or evidence of silicone material. Cross-sections fail to reveal any solid or nodular densities or evidence of tumor.

Specimen K is a combination of silicone saline mammary implant. No specific identifying stamps or marks are present. **It appears intact although the outer envelope is devoid of fluid.** It weighs 220 gm. and measures up to 13 cm in diameter.

The implant was missing 110 gm. of fluid from the final numbers upon insertion eleven years previously. What happened to the silicon? Was it reabsorbed? Did it dissolve? Why is there no fluid in the outer envelope of the sac?

The second time I was diagnosed with breast cancer, it was a totally different experience. The shock was not as great as I had been living with the "BIG C" for eleven years by then. I also knew a lot more about the disease and what it takes o survive. What I was not ready for was how much harder it was physically this time. Granted I was eleven years older, the drugs were stronger, and the anesthesia better, but I was really sick.

There is a reason they call the chemotherapy drug, Adriamycin, the "Red Devil." Adriamycin takes you to hell and back. The anti-nausea pills and medicine helped with the initial infusion of medicine but did nothing for the twelve hours later when the "devil" came to visit.

I remember one night in particular after treatment. I must admit it is a foggy memory, but I remember shaking in my hands, then violently shaking on the bed. My husband lay on top of me to keep me in bed and prevent me from hurting myself. What a scare that was for him, and what fear our bodies can create for us when our bodies are out of control.

After several doses of chemotherapy of different levels and kinds, my tolerance for the drug war was abating. I knew there were a few things worse than dying of cancer. Not living my life the way I wanted to live it was my greater concern.

Do not get me wrong, I like life, even with all its complications and disappointments, but there are ways I have chosen to live. When my hands and feet began to be numb more often than they had feeling, I knew I had to make some decisions. My hobbies mainly included my hands and feet.

Could I live without playing the piano, hiking, and writing? The things I loved to do mostly required my fingers and my toes to function. I did not want to have "life" at the expense of being myself. I did not even have a particular kind of reconstruction because it would affect my hobbies.

I decided to stop taking the drug Taxol, as it seemed to affect my extremities after only two months. When I lived in Switzerland, I started hiking and continued whenever and wherever I could. It is hard enough to climb hills and mountains and go long distances, but with no feeling in my toes, it would have been miserable.

I had numbness in my hands, probably caused by carrying a backpack and having limited lymph nodes under my armpits. If you want to find a breast cancer survivor hiker, look for the ones with their hands over their heads. It helps with the draining of lymph back into the body. Wearing a backpack can cut off the circulation around the arm area, and we must move our extremities.

My cancer support group met for years later, and when we would hike, someone always had her hands over her head at any one time. I am sure it looks strange, but it works. No one had the potential side effect of breast surgery, lymphedema or swelling of the arms.

The piano had been a part of my life since I was five years old. I was not good enough with short stubby fingers to be professional, but I was a good hobby pianist. I even did "gigs" and was paid. Numbness in my hands made them slow and tingling. As a pianist, I do like to make those eighty-eight piano keys work with all those ten fingers. I quit Taxol for good when my hands went numb.

The physicians were concerned, and family and friends thought I was crazy, but I could not live without hiking, piano playing, and writing in my journal. Was it the right decision? Who knows? Now, I am decades past the last breast cancer. I still have numbness in my fingers when I type, or after playing the piano for more than thirty minutes. But I can hike three miles before the numbness in my toe begins. It was the right choice for me.

These are more medical reports after moving to Colorado Springs.

Penrose — St. Francis Colorado Springs Radiology

4/20/99 (6 months after a second breast cancer diagnosis)

> Mammograms of left breast were obtained from Texas Women's Imaging, dated 18 September 1998. These were used for comparison with the current study of 20 April 1999. The mass and abnormal microcalcifications, which were noted in the upper outer left breast on the previous study, are absent. The current examination shows NO evidence of breast malignancy.

Penrose Cancer Center — Physician Notes 5/99

Outpatient Radiation Oncology

History of Present Illness:

> The patient has a prior history of a right breast carcinoma treated in July of 1987 with mastectomy. Subsequently, reconstruction with silicone implant resulted in rupture and eventually; the patient had a saline implant placed.

ALLERGIES:

> Sulfa, Tetracycline, Ampicillin, Cipro, and Erythromycin

I began the six weeks of radiation therapy after I recovered from my last chemotherapy. Daily for five days a week, I drove downtown about twenty minutes, parked the car, and walked to the oncology center. They had placed a small tattoo where the tumor had been and used that purple dot to line up the radiation tubes for treatment. The whole process took about fifteen minutes after the first visit.

I remember the tiredness setting in after four weeks of daily radiation. But after the exhaustion I had felt over my last two years working, it was nothing. I was not working, so I slept, read, walked a bit each day and ate good healthy food.

I wanted a long life, but not at the cost of quality of life. Hiking was the first thing I did after my last radiation treatment. I yearned to give myself nature's healing gifts.

The radiation therapy team said to me, "Treatment is over, go out and live your life."

Chapter 5

Second Implant

When I am fighting an illness, trying to make the right decisions for myself, I demand that my support team respects my decisions. I never considered not replacing my ruptured silicone implant with a saline implant, but I do not remember even having a discussion about options. As it is said, "life is not a dress rehearsal, it is the final act." Keep moving and fighting to live. The new job started only two months after I finished radiation treatment, but I had not worked for over a year and we needed money.

In 2000, according to complete cosmetic surgery procedures statistics of American Society of Plastic Surgeons in 2020, 212,500 women had breast augmentation, including approximately 100,000 breast cancer reconstruction, often with implants. This overall number would increase by 48 percent in 2018 to 313,735 women and teenagers having breast enlargements with silicone or saline implants. This staggering number includes saline implants, which first required and received approval in 2000, and silicone gel implants approved by the FDA in 2006.

Journal

Summer 1999

June 6, 1999

I went on my first hike with my friend Gaye. We went to Cutler Trai in Colorado Springs and climbed 400 feet in one mile. Up and down a different path at Seven Falls and then climbing back up to Helen Hun Falls in Cheyenne Canyon. Only three miles and I am tired. After six week of radiation and months of chemotherapy, I can still hike, but it is really draining.

I am looking at what supplements I need to heal. What changes do make in eating? I am trying a homeopathic fast with vegetable juices an protein powders. I have been eating juice and veggies for three days an feel nauseous in the morning. My body is purging itself of radiation an chemotherapy side effects. (I now know, I was also getting rid of silicone i my body from the ruptured implant.)

June 17, 1999

Detoxing takes time. Nausea, period, low energy, and sleeping nine plu hours. I did a sauna and hot bath, foot rub and skin cleansing with Epson salts in the bath. Drinking lots of water and teas with no caffeine and n dairy and still multiple bowel movements per day. It is not hard to detoxify but it is like going through chemotherapy again with the nausea.

My headache is very intense and has been for two days. The fog in m brain was severe and only lessened with sleep and a walk. I need to be alon as this is too hard to do around other people.

June 19, 1999

Day 6 of the homeopathic fast. I did my first coffee enema yesterday an another today. It is awkward but not painful. I did feel better and had mucl more energy. My anxiety was high and I felt like I was in the "pit" of the fast I feel like the toxins are being released.

My joints all hurt, my period is weird and I did not have herpes. M liver and gallbladder really hurt today. After the grapefruit juice with lemo and oranges brew, laying on my right side, and then an enema, the pain i gone. Another coffee enema today and I try to be kind to myself learnin; the technique. The goal is to hold it inside for fifteen minutes, but crampin; makes it difficult. Detoxing takes so much time.

June 22, 1999

Discovering purpose in this time of recovery is my goal. I want to tell my story and how God has brought me here for such a time as this.

My detox weeks are over. Bowels are loose, but I am adding acidophilus and am back on grain, rice, and tofu for protein. I feel better, cleansed and eat much less. I think I will have to adjust to never having dairy again.

Nine months ago, my whole life changed. It is good to feel hope to survive.

Lord, thank you for these six months of increasing health and good changes.

July 7, 1999

Twelve years ago today, I was diagnosed with breast cancer the first time. The cleansing is working to clear my body of chemotherapy and radiation toxins. My energy is better and I am sleeping eight hours. I had a massage and the masseuse felt I had really detoxed myself, as I no longer had lumps in my upper body. I had a slight headache and much gas from another detox with multiple bowel movements. When I start counting bowel movements, I need a job.

July 18, 1999

I am fighting diarrhea, swollen neck glands, and small herpes and want the illness to be gone. I started talk therapy and this will not be pleasant. My books and readings on healing include John Wimber, founder of Vineyard USA. He said, "Healing can take so much time and we do not know why." Healing takes place in stages: 1. Pain leaves; 2. Impairment departs; 3. Disfigurement of the structure takes more time; 4. Rest afterward.

August 24, 1999

I went through the first day of my new job with an internal net over my brain. The brain fog got worse in the afternoon after baked potato with meat, cheese, and sour cream. Things I am allergic to for sure and it was too much. The wrong food, like carbohydrates and dairy, affect my memory. I bet I get herpes from it as well.

August 29, 1999

My new oncologist in Denver called regarding the estrogen status of the tumor and wants to discuss treatment options differently. My former doctor in Colorado Springs "has his notes full of erroneous information." I feel my anger again to the medical personnel but want to experience forgiveness and grace.

Fall 1999

September 15, 1999

My tiredness does seem physical now. I have brain fog and was in bed almost eleven hours. The tiredness seems spiritual? Physical? Mental? I do not think I am depressed, but all the symptoms are there. My neck hurts in the cool and damp weather. I think my body is fighting something. God, please not cancer again.

The anti-parasite stuff seems to be working. I have increased my fruits and vegetables but have limited motivation. Now! Go! Walk outside for twenty minutes. Get up and go!

September 17, 1999

I am definitely fearful of the pain and the herpes. I am so tired on this trip to Dallas and my feet just ache. My headache overwhelms me. Every night I take a muscle relaxer because there is no downtime to relax from work.

October 4, 1999

I have tightness and pain in my left neck. Is it from surgery? I have been stretching and meditating for an hour to recover. I have had two falls and with my lack of upper body exercise, is that the reason?

It has been hard the last two weeks with the one-year anniversary of my second cancer. One year ago, I had the first lumpectomy and implant replacement. Maybe my shock was the only way I got through it.

I am delaying the mammogram. My breast feels fine but with hot flashes, sore throat, and clumsiness, I hope to get better and yet it never happens. The knee herpes is worse. I must look at all these problems, as I just cannot become totally well.

October 8, 1999

My cold has been released and my nose is running and my throat is sore. The fever is gone. It has been a year since my last awful cold after surgery.

November 20, 1999

I am in St. Louis, Missouri, my husband is in Ft. Worth, Texas, and our home is in Colorado Springs, Colorado, a normal weekend for us. We had sex before I left, which was the first time since April.

Winter 1999-2000

December 4, 1999

I am sad and scared, because of the amount of rest required to recover from travel. On top of the neck pain, irregular periods, and a migraine, no wonder I crave sleep. The neck pain sometimes goes up on the scale to a six or seven out of ten for days.

Though I get sick again
Though I am alone
Though my husband never gets a job,
Yet I will trust the Lord.

December 21, 1999

It is the first illness in five weeks. I am fighting a cold, flu, herpes, and fever. The cold is mild with only one herpes lesion and great pain. Could I still be healing from last year? With all the supplements, vitamins, rest, and eating right, life has to get better. There is no choice. The pain is hard to bear sometimes, but when God says I am done, I will leave.

Lord, may Your hand be on my head. May You guide my actions. Give my family contentment as they come closer to You. As the song says, "Take my life and let it be, consecrated Lord to Thee." Take my hands and feet and lead me in Your ways as we begin a New Millennium.

February 2, 2000

I thought I had allergies, but it has turned into a cold with a severe sore throat and now head congestion and cough. Now there is no sleep because I cannot breathe. Diarrhea, flu, two periods, fever, exhaustion, food poisoning, and constipation have occurred in the last five weeks.

I am worried about my lack of health and all the effects it has on me. How do I connect my mind and body to greater health? Influenza can be as life threatening as my cancer because I am allergic to most antibiotics. So if flu turns to bacterial pneumonia, there is nothing to be done. I visited the emergency room for medication. Is a true act of bravery in 2000 to take care of our health, and then take care of work?

February 29, 2000

I went to see a chiropractor that told me I had seven vertebrae out of place. I realize how much pain I live with in my back. My gut empties out with diarrhea from fast from any food color and eating only white rice and cauliflower. My nausea has been high and it reminds me of my detox time.

Summer 2000

June 1, 2000

Diarrhea is back and I see the gastroenterologist today. Is there ever a time when my health will be constant? I can finally run after four years with no pain. I can breathe rhythmically and I am recovering.

June 10, 2000

I am slipping again into the darkness. It comes over my soul and I beat back the grayness amid the beauty of what I see. I know today, I must feel the sadness, the loss, and depression sweeping into my heart.

Depression came after the emergency landing in Memphis from Houston. I called my husband and my parents from the airplane phone and said "good-bye and I love you." I had forty minutes of quiet as we slowly descended with one engine and watched the Mississippi Delta spread out in front of me.

When the pilot banked the plane slowly, there were no planes on the runway or near us in the air. Emergency vehicles lined the runway. I said prayers for the pilot and his crew, as we prepared to land, flip, spin, or burn…. We bounced so hard that I held myself into the seat.

Applause erupted as he finally slowed the plane, and shaking consumed my body, as I know this is only an experience survived by a few. In fifteen years, the pilot and stewardess had never had that experience.

Near-death experiences for the fourth time in a week: my friend with cancer, my husband with cancer, rattlesnake on the hike, and now near fatal plane ride.

June 11, 2000

The "gorilla" came out of my closet to sit on my chest today and smothered my joy of being alive. That is what depression feels like to me. I sobbed at a song, had no smile on my face, and then sadness descended, blotting out me as the little girl in that plane. No one who has not experienced that kind of descent can realize how scary and helpless you feel. I can act normal, but the gorilla sits, watches, and waits. Today the gorilla visited, and I have not been out of bed. I have no energy for anything that gives me joy.

I cannot even remember my own phone number. My brain has seized up and overloaded. I cannot function. I want to die. The last two years of illness and the additional stress of the last two weeks and I have nothing left in reserves. I feel so alone without friends, without love, and without God. The mental and emotional effects spill into every area of my life.

June 14, 2000

The drugs I took for my constant diarrhea caused the deep depression, so now the doctor put me on a different drug for my gut and added an anti-depressant to the mix. I was getting better within twelve hours off the medication. I will take diarrhea over the depression.

Fall 2001

September 4, 2001

On the road trip through Kansas, hot flashes, herpes from heat, diarrhea was so bad I had two accidents along the road. I think it was the food on the trip.

September 11, 2001

The world changed on 9/11/01.

Before terrorism
After clouded skies change us
Forever.
The towers crumble

After errant flights change us
Forever.
Air highways
After terror on the ground changes us
Forever.
People scared
Unexplained violence changes us
Forever.
We go home
After calls to family and friends
And grieve and change us
Forever and Forever.

I saw the Pentagon and it is in shambles with the war zone effect. All business has stopped as we stay by the phone and TV. We all want to be connected, get gas in our car, money, food stocked, as it is an act of war. The F15 and F16 jet fighters are checking out the air space in Colorado Springs for safety for NORAD. Tears and sorrow use up our emotion over the next few days. Work is minimal as we are in shock as a country.

September 12, 2001

The nightmare is real. I awoke to see five Arabs identified and no flights are allowed in from Europe. I heard the C30 cargo plane lumbering low over the house in Colorado Springs. The five military bases are all closed; access to the water supply is closed. Barges full of body bags are crossing to New Jersey. Semi-trucks are there to take away the dead. Papers from the World Trade Center are found up to three miles away.

I would awake and see that plane crashing into the building. Surely this is not real but a dream. There is nothing to compare. Hospitals prepare for the injuries, but no one comes. Colorado F16 Air Guard patrols the skies all night long.

My boss drives to Colorado from Dallas as the flight was canceled. Our work colleagues in New York are driving home to Seattle, trying to get away from the toxic chaos in New York. Our chief financial officer for the new company that bought us was on one of the planes.

The decisions of mundane things of work pale in comparison to the real events. If I could only sleep through the night....

September 17, 2001,

The hole and rip in my soul mirror everyone's. I wake up, stop, catch my breath, and know my world is changed. I cry hysterically at additional bad news and am honored and inspired by my countrymen.

The world is united in prayer and dependence on God for wisdom, blessings, and justice. We look to God as the source of answers in a questioning world.

> "He who binds to himself a joy,
> Does the winged life destroy.
> He who kisses a joy as it flies,
> Lives in eternity's sunrise."
> ~"Eternity" by William Blake

October 15, 2001

We are flying to Washington, DC to meet the directors of Medicaid about our product. It is a crazy time to fly. Hazmat trucks are coming to greet our isolated silver tube. White powder has left residue on a suitcase. After anthrax scares, no one takes any chances. A silly young college kid is escorted off the plane and met by law enforcement.

We all look around at people suspiciously on our plane. Finding the buff, short hair men with a jacket on in the exit row reveals the air marshals. A late boarder on the plane hands a suspiciously light computer into the scared witless stewardess's hands. There is a "hole" in the Pentagon.

October 23, 2001

My neck hurts so badly that I went for a massage, which led me to a chiropractor that diagnosed: 1. Virus settling in neck; 2. Heart meridian is stressed; 3. Adrenal glands are stressed; 4. Cystic valve is immune depressed. What does it mean?

November 5, 2001

I have been sick for three weeks. I am sure I am fighting strep throat but am allergic to all antibiotics. My fever returns regularly and I feel crummy.

Winter 2001-2002

December 3, 2001

We went to a Christmas tree farm to get a tree. My head is stuffed up and must be allergens to two trees in the house. God, please help me, I am miserable in this world. I have coughed and blown my nose for seven weeks! Please, God? Give me a good day sometimes as I have forgotten what they are like and this contributes to my hopelessness.

January 24, 2002

San Jose, California. I am very sick. I drank tea and ate oatmeal, blueberry muffins, and chocolate espresso and had a strong reaction. Then massive cramping and diarrhea followed before I boarded the plane home. I felt like throwing up any moment on the plane ride, and think I have food poisoning.

Why was I in another exhausting job that caused me to have multiple illnesses and yet keep going? The answer is simple. Money. Lots of it. The Internet dot. com boom was happening, and I was in a high-tech company selling into that commercial area. I was their lead salesperson in healthcare, and selling intranets to Fortune 500 companies was a blast. We had a good product, I had wonderful colleagues, and a great boss.

I am a long-term survivor of two different breast cancers: one at the age of thirty and a different kind of breast cancer eleven years later at the age of forty-one. I survived, and did many alternative and, to some people, strange things to help me physically, mentally, spiritually, and emotionally heal from cancer and chemotherapy.

No one ever said anything about silicone toxicity or healing from a leaking breast implant. There were many non-medical things I did to improve my health during my cancers, treatment, and recovery.

Chapter 6

Alternative Therapies for Healing

A lternative therapies allowed me to actively contribute something to improving my health and hopefully living longer. Here are some more things I did to heal from chemotherapy, radiation treatment, and the ruptured silicone implant. I drank bottled water and ate mostly organic food and continue to this day to prepare most of my food at home.

Exercise

Exercise every day and when possible, do it outside. I was sometimes so sick and weak, I could only walk down the steps, around the house, and back upstairs. This is giving your body what I call "live messages." As I healed, I went on long hikes. After I completed six weeks of radiation, I walked six miles the following day with two friends. I did it, but I slept for the next two days.

I am an exercise and fresh air fanatic and even walked outside every day in Colorado's winter during chemotherapy and radiation. For me, three miles walking daily is ideal, and I change exercising to include weight training, elliptical and other climbing machines. My exercise regimen has changed with aging, but I still exercise three to four times per week.

Energy Healing

I visited an "energy" healer every month for two years post-treatment. She would ask me each time, "Now, you pray to Jesus right? Do you pray to the dolphins or angels or anything else?" What? She was weird, but I was willing to try anything. She would lay different vials of herbs on my chest and then raise my arm and see if my muscles would reject the vial by how easy it was to push down my arm. This is muscle testing and is not approved by the medical establishment.

Massage and Reflexology

Reflexology and massage monthly keep me in touch with my body, allow me to feel better, and cleanse all the toxins that went to the bottom of my feet and throughout my system. I had reflexology. "Reflexology is the practice of applying pressure to the feet and hands, utilizing specific thumb, finger, and hand techniques without the use of oil, cream, or lotion. It is based on a system of zones and reflex areas that reflect an image of the body on the feet and hands with a premise that such work effects a physical change in the body."[2]

I had a regular massage and added raindrop therapy. Raindrop therapy is a healing technique using pure essential oils. "Raindrop therapy combines aromatherapy, reflexology, massage, and moist heat to create healing and cleansing through structural and electrical alignment to the body. The purpose of the therapy is to bring total balance, harmony, and body wellness, including, mental, physical, and emotional."[3]

Detoxification

I had detoxification cleansing of the blood, liver, and colon for years, including my famous post-radiation coffee enemas. "Detoxification is the process of clearing toxins from the body or neutralizing or transforming them and clearing excess mucus and congestion."[4]

Nutritional Healing

I met a dietitian from Colorado Springs, Colorado, Diana Dyer, M.S., R.D., CNSD, who had cancer three times: a neuroblastoma as a child and two different breast cancers. I bought her booklet, which told the story of her cancer and her change in eating habits.

As my support group friend Laura said, "I have eaten broccoli all my life and now I have cancer. What else can I do?"

Diana had a list of things to consider in her booklet *A Dietitian's Cancer Story*.
- Maintain a healthy weight for your height and exercise regularly.
- Reduce or eliminate alcohol.
- Increase fiber with 6 servings of whole-grain foods, 2 servings of legumes

and 5–9 colorful fruits and vegetables.

- Reduce fat in your diet to around 20% of calories by avoiding fat substitutes, using only extra-virgin olive oil or canola oil, use butter not margarine, lean meats and reduce portion size.
- Consume soy products 3 servings a day because of their anti-carcinogenic compounds.
- Use only reduced-fat dairy products 1% and low-fat yogurt.
- Limit grilled, broiled and blackened meats and fish because it can create carcinogens.
- Use flax seed with every meal.

I had done many of these things like being a vegetarian for twenty years, so I did not have much change in my diet. I have continued to do most of these things (except I do not like flax seed) for the last twenty years. After my second cancer, I could not seem to get enough protein without meat, so I did reintroduce meat and fish into my diet. I have maintained small portions of meat and eat organic when possible.

Getting nine helpings of fruit and vegetables a day does require creative cooking and planning. Shakes, dried fruit, juices (without sugar), salads, dried cranberries, kebabs of vegetables; stir-fried vegetables make it simple to increase your intake.

During chemotherapy for the second breast cancer, I knew I needed help from someone who could help me fight the "medicine" with nutrition. I called my friend Abby, a nutritionist, and asked her to come and cook for me for a few days. This was no easy task I was asking her to do as she had small twins, work, and husband to care for as well.

But Abby came, and I have told her many times she saved my life with kale and dill. She went to the store and bought me organic potatoes, healthy broth, expensive fresh dill, and organic kale. She cut everything in small pieces and cooked them slowly. At first, I could only eat the broth, but within a day, my appetite was returning, at least for her concoction. It was the first meal I had eaten in two weeks, and cut up kale and potatoes remain a favorite of mine to this day.

Emotional Healing

When I first saw Dr. Bernie Siegel's book *Love, Medicine, and Miracles*[5] after my first cancer diagnosis, I thumbed through the copy at a bookstore. Dr. Siegel was a medical doctor who primarily treated cancer patients. He wanted to understand why some people survived their diagnosis, and others died quietly and quickly from the exact same diagnosis.

He began to research how emotions affected the survival of cancers and how emotional health had actually impacted those who received a diagnosis. I remember reading the book while standing in the aisle and finding out about a person with breast cancer saying, "I had to get something off my chest." Bingo! This resonated true with my own breast cancer, but it would be over a decade before I understood this revelation. "I encourage my patients to have faith in God, but not to expect Him (Her) to do all the work," says Dr. Bernie Siegel.

I bought a set of cassette tapes (remember this was in 1987) of healing meditations that Bernie Siegel had recorded. I also started recording my dreams and even tried drawing pictures in my journal regarding the cancer experience.

One example in the book or tape was seeing cancer cells as Pac Man bubbles. Then Pac Man would eat the floating cells whenever the person was having chemotherapy. He advised us to pick our own visual and to use it throughout the chemotherapy. I chose a beautiful white horse galloping through a field stamping down the cancer cells. Since a horse had started all my travails, this visual was ironic. I would trace the chemotherapy in my mind through my port in my chest throughout the body, therefore befriending the medication and giving it an extra boost to kill the cancer cells.

I used Dr. Siegel's guided meditations after treatment was over and saw myself on a professional stage. The audience was made up of people I loved. Some were alive and others had died. I remember being completely naked on the stage with my scarred breast and saying, "I have to stop performing for everyone else. I want to live!"

I found an old newspaper column from the humorist Dave Berry, "She's Home and Feeling Better Now." It is a description of the hospital experience from the eyes of an uninformed layperson. The article portrays the hospital food, staples in his wife, and a drain as the reason she was now so sick, when she looked fine upon arrival.

I believe the whole cancer experience has to include recognizing the doses of humor in the drama in order to thrive, not just survive. The importance of joy and humor is not to be underestimated. When is the last time you laughed hysterically during an illness?

One person told me, "Someday, our descendants will look back on this time of cancer treatment like we look at people using leeches to draw out impurities in the past centuries. We cut, poison, and give radiation to people who are already sick. How crazy is that?"

I learned to take myself less seriously but appreciate more beauty. I began to eally live in the "moments to remember." Have I failed to always live this way? Of course, but there are a few statements I share with anyone facing a radical lifestyle change due to their health.

- If you had only six months to live, would you be doing what you are doing now? If yes, praise God. If not, what would you change? I suggest they make those changes as quickly as they can.
- Do you have a bucket list? What dates do you want to achieve it? I put together a bucket list of things I wanted to achieve and by perseverance and God's gracious gifts to me, I completed them all within the next thirty years.
  - A house with a picket fence
  - A dog
  - Hiking in all fifty states
  - Riding an elephant and camel in the countries where they live (China and Egypt)
  - Pay off my house mortgage by the time I am sixty-two
  - Have a substantial savings account when I retire
  - Write and publish a book
- Why do you think you have this disease? What are you learning from this experience? Get a therapist or a good friend who will listen to you as you go through the journey.
- God did not create human "doings." He created human beings, so how can you begin to shift from a doing to a being?
- Every ache and pain will have a different connotation for you after cancer treatment. It is what I call "toe cancer." It is perfectly normal.

I say to the newly diagnosed breast cancer person, "You are not going to die next week, and probably will be alive next year. Breathe." I also tell them, "Whatever you choose as your treatment, I will support you." If people in your life do not support your decisions, get them out of your life! One of my family members who had recurrent breast cancer in her early thirties remarked on the changes I had made in my eating when she visited. She said to me, "If I have to eat like that (healthy), I would rather die." And she did, within eighteen months. I supported her decision on not changing her food and nutrition.

A friend took hormonal therapy after her cancer, no chemotherapy, and one dose of radiation, but nothing else. I support her decision. Another friend treated her Stage 4 metastatic breast cancer with a not-yet-FDA-approved treatment from Germany, which required her to fly to California many times to receive therapy.

I support her decision. Another woman had lumpectomy surgery and did nothing else. I support her decision.

The lesson for the medical profession from my support group was: "If anything helps the nausea be less, the healthy white cell count to stay high, and to aid my progress positively through treatment, support it!"

Kitchen Table Wisdom: Stories that Heal, by Rachel Naomi Remen, MD, was a book I found after my second breast cancer in 1998. She was an early pioneer in the mind/body health field. Through her compilation of stories of patients, I deepened my commitment to understanding the connection of my own mind and emotions to my cancer. I learned that we tend to not discuss our death, pain, and suffering, but when we talk about these things, there is healing in our words. If I held these words inside me, and did not discuss it openly, the words would harm me. I would read, identify, process, and go to the next story in her book. I still read the book over twenty years later.

Grace and Grit: Spirituality and Healing in the Life and Death of Treya Killam Wilber, by Ken Wilber, was a source of deeper knowledge for me. It tells the story of Treya who had breast cancer and subsequently dies. Treya was in a support group led by Dr. Rachel Remen at her clinic in Sausalito, California. Dr. Remen is the author of the above-mentioned book, Kitchen Table Wisdom.

Grace and Grit taught me about many spiritual and emotional practices I was not familiar with at the time. I believe we can learn from anyone who has gone through the illness or disease process regardless of his or her faith, ethnic, or socioeconomic background.

This book spoke to my heart and my emotions. People wanted to believe that I had beaten cancer, I was cured, and it was over. I believed I had "failed" by getting sick. Whether I was thinking I had caused the illness, allowed the illness, or benefited from cancer, there was guilt and a sense of failure. My emotions were not healthy or steady during cancer, and I was thankful to have another young woman or a support group of breast cancer survivors to discuss the experience.

Therapy or counseling can benefit everyone. I believe that telling someone about all your crazy experiences are very beneficial to the healing of a serious disease. Their job is not to be emotionally involved and to therapeutically listen to us. Our emotions have a way of telling us what is going on in our physical bodies.

I went to a psychologist many years post-cancer who helped me heal through Eye Movement Desensitization and Reprocessing (EMDR). EMDR is an integrative psychotherapy approach that has been extensively researched and proven effective for the treatment of trauma. EMDR is a set of standardized protocols that ncorporates elements from many treatment approaches.

Therapists helped me to identify my sadness, grief, anger, and hope. There is a inancial cost to this, but for me, it has been worth it. I am very thankful to all my lifferent therapists throughout the years, and I go for a "tune-up" every few years ust as I go see my primary care doctor annually for a wellness check.

Chapter 7

Spiritual Healing

My survival has been miraculous. I have known an equal amount of people who survived and did not survive cancer. I ask myself and God regularly, "Why am I still alive and he/she is not?" God has still not answered me two decades after breast cancer number two.

I had one whole year of my relative physical health. But slowly, I began to get sicker again in 2002. The year also included my husband's prostate cancer diagnosis and treatment, purchase of a new house, and introduction of a Brittany spaniel into our home. It was a difficult year, and my recollections through my journal are of marital challenges, work travel, and successes.

My emotional health suffered during this time, and I turned more to God for hope in the midst of this constant sickness. God had always been a part of my life and during my cancers; I had turned to Him and the Bible more and more.

If anyone says they go through a serious illness or trauma and do not have a crisis or questions about their faith, they are either delusional or people of extraordinary belief.

I was somewhere in-between by questioning God for the reasons I was always sick, and wondering what good was coming out of this crisis. Speaking as a person who is a Christ-follower, the spiritual healing of my soul was a deep part of a transformational process.

Before I was thrown off the horse and ruptured my first breast implant, I had gone through breast cancer and a painful divorce after finding out I needed to be tested for AIDS. My twelve-year marriage was severed as if my arm was cut of with no anesthesia and I was dripping blood from the wound.

I could not believe that the man of faith I married, the man who was my best friend, the man who verbally abused me at times, was questioning his sexuality. tell the story of those first three months after the revelation in my book *Deception Revelation to Release*.

I had relocated to Indiana to be nearer my family as I recovered from five difficult years. My faith was central to my core being, and I had had spiritual experiences that grounded me in the truth of God and the love of Jesus. I identified with Christ' suffering, and believed I would see "good in the land of the living again."

The decline of my health, once again in my late thirties, was not a good time Even though I was practicing healthy spiritual disciplines such as prayer, scripture reading, meditating, and worshiping with other believers, I was fearful I had cancer again. I recognized that my health was in a very precarious state.

I was practicing good nutrition, running daily for exercise and stress relief Regular massage, cranial sacral treatment, and nutritional supplements were routine. I had friends, both old and new in my life and an active social life. My career was soaring, and I was able to use my skills to improve healthcare in the surrounding communities by bringing additional specialists to rural areas of Indiana, Illinois, and Kentucky.

I joined a divorce recovery group to better understand and receive from others deep healing through teaching, discussion, and fun activities. No longer was I involved in teaching the Bible weekly to large groups of women. There were smaller groups of Bible studies I joined for short times and seasons. I was not listening to God at this time in my life, but I was having fun.

A few years later, at forty-one years old, eleven years after my first breast cancer, I said, "If I am going to be this sick, I do not want to live." I was asking God to go ahead and let me come to Him. Sickness affected my spiritual life. I did not even think about breast implant illness, even though I had ruptured my silicon implant.

After the second breast cancer and after the silicone implant was replaced with a saline implant, I was physically well, and growing in my spiritual closeness to God. Unfortunately, I divorced again and became increasingly sick eight years after the replacement implant, and I prayed again to not be here on earth. My second round of breast implant illness (BII) began at this time and continued for another decade of increasing illness. I lived on the knife-edge of disease and was confused and inconsolable.

Several books impacted me greatly during my times of sickness and healing.

Authors and their stories in books were my sources of inspiration, healing, and hope.

My Bible is filled with dates and notations of verses that gave me comfort during the surgeries, illnesses, and recoveries. I started marking my Bible with dates and words on July 7, 1987, and praying for strength with these verses.

> "For this reason, I bow my knees before the Father, from whom every family in heaven and on earth derives its name, that He would grant you, according to the riches of His glory, to be strengthened with power through His Spirit in the inner man, so that Christ may dwell in your hearts through faith; and that you, being rooted and grounded in love, may be able to comprehend with all the saints what is the breadth and length and height and depth, and to know the love of Christ which surpasses knowledge, that you may be filled up to all the fullness of God.
>
> Now to Him who is able to do far more abundantly beyond all that we ask or think, according to the power that works within us, to Him be the glory in the church and in Christ Jesus to all generations forever and ever. Amen." Ephesians 3:14–21 (NASB)

A man at my church gave me an unknown scripture the month after my first cancer diagnosis. I had never heard it before and I did not know the person very well. This scripture was an exceptional gift. I have memorized it and share it with other people who are struggling with anything.

> "Do not fear, for I am with you; Do not anxiously look about you, for I am your God. I will strengthen you, surely I will help you, Surely I will uphold you with My righteous right hand." Isaiah 41:10 (NASB)

I wrote, "I am sick!" beside the following psalm in my Bible. Anti-nausea medication has helped people so much and yet, I was putting toxic medication into my system to kill fast-growing cells.

> "I cry aloud with my voice to the LORD; I make supplication with my voice to the LORD. I pour out my complaint before Him; I declare my trouble before Him. When my spirit was overwhelmed within me, You knew my path. In the way where I walk, They have hidden a trap for me." Psalm 142: 1–3 (NASB)

When I was ill, people of good meaning and faith said stupid things. They asked me, "Do you have enough faith? Are you praying for healing? Is there sin in your life you have not repented of?" I truly wanted to scream at these well-meaning people who do not know what to say to someone so young and so sick.

I read books during my diagnosis, treatment, and recovery time, and they had a great impact on my life of faith. Charles R. Swindoll and his books allowed me to explore grace. I did not come from a faith background that emphasized the grace of God. I had been raised with being a "good girl" and that what I did would keep me close to God. The focus of my faith was more about what I did than about what Jesus had done for me already. There was a poem included in the book *The Grace Awakening* by Charles R Swindoll, which I copied into my journal and read often.

"Letting Go"
Author unknown

To "let go" does not mean to stop caring;
it means I can't do it for someone else.

To "let go" is not to cut myself off,
it's the realization I can't control another.

To "let go" is not to enable,
but to allow learning from natural consequences.

To "let go" is to admit powerlessness,
which means the outcome is not in my hands.

To "let go" is not to try to change or blame another;
it's to make the most of myself.

To "let go" is not to care for,
but to care about.

To "let go" is not to fix,
but to be supportive.

To "let go" is not to judge,
but to allow another to be a human being.

To "let go" is not to be in the middle arranging the outcomes,
but to allow others to affect their own destinies.

To "let go" is not to be protective;
it's to permit another to face reality.

To "let go" is not to deny,
but to accept.

To "let go" is not to nag, scold or argue,
but instead to search out my own shortcomings, and correct them.

To "let go" is not to adjust everything to my desires
but to take each day as it comes,
and cherish myself in it.

To "let go" is not to criticize and regulate anybody
but to try to become what I dream I can be.

To "let go" is not to regret the past,
but to grow and live for the future.

To "let go" is to fear less,
and love more.

Scripture was important to me after I returned from living in Switzerland for three years. I was not yet sick from my silicone implant. I was thankful I had lived five years after my breast cancer diagnosis.

"For You formed my inward parts; You wove me in my mother's womb. I will give thanks to You, for I am fearfully and wonderfully made; Wonderful are Your works, and my soul knows it very well." Psalm 139:13–14 (NASB)

Another book I read was *The Tapestry* by Edith Schaeffer. She was married to theologian Francis Schaeffer and recorded his life and works in this memoir. They had started L'Abri, a spiritual retreat in Switzerland, as a place to come and ask hard questions regarding faith. I had visited L'Abri during my time in Switzerland after I experienced cancer, depression, infertility, and marital challenges. My faith was shaky at times, and her words comforted me that God was big enough to handle all my questions.

"Never do I cease to marvel, as I thank God for Franky (her husband), that He is indeed an all-powerful, all-wise God whom we can trust with the overall pattern of 'The Tapestry.'" pg. 348[6]

Her husband Francis was diagnosed with cancer and she writes these words.

"How does one pray at such a time? Does one make it just begging to have the illness taken away? pg. 615

Edith Schaeffer refers to the story of Jesus healing the lame man in John 5:1–15 when Jesus asked the beggar "Do you wish to get well?" And later Jesus says to the man, "Behold, you have become well; do not sin anymore, so that nothing worse happens to you."

Dealing with the necessary spiritual healing of my soul was as important as the emotional, nutritional, physical healing that followed my cancers and subsequent breast implant illness. I am bold to say, it was the most important healing I experienced. Reading *The Tapestry* gave me hope that my suffering would have meaning someday. The picture of the beautiful tapestry of our lives as seen from above does not show all the mistakes, loose threads and incomplete parts that are visible from the backside. The meaning of these experiences would not be revealed as I was facing these things, but someday I would understand. God was weaving a beautiful tapestry full of bright colors and hope.

During dark days and nights of battles to stay alive after cancer, I found scriptures that spoke to the "enemy" of disease were of great solace and hope.

. "O our God, will You not judge them? For we are powerless before this great multitude who are coming against us; nor do we know what to do, but our eyes are on You." 2 Chronicles 20:12 (NASB)

"I would have despaired unless I had believed that I would see the goodness of the LORD In the land of the living. Wait for the LORD; Be strong and let your heart take courage; Yes, wait for the LORD." Psalm 27:13–14 (NASB)

During my second divorce, a friend shared this with me and I still use it when I am overwhelmed with illness or do not know what to do. I am His creation and God knows my name. What a comfort that is to me, and to all the people who struggle with feeling unseen, unheard, and unknown.

"But now, thus says the LORD, your Creator, O Jacob, And He who formed you, O Israel, "Do not fear, for I have redeemed you; I have called you by name; you are Mine!" Isaiah 43:1 (NASB)

I was scared often about my poor health. I was depressed, scared, and confused, and I used the promise below from Zechariah. God's chosen people in Judah and

Israel had turned away from the Lord Almighty. He had told them through the prophet Zechariah to "Administer true justice, show mercy and compassion" (7:9 NIV), and yet they had refused to pay attention. I wanted God to know I was sorry or repentant for anything I had done to cause these diseases, even though I did not think I had caused it myself.

> "So I will save you that you may become a blessing. Do not fear; let your hands be strong." Zechariah 8:13b (NASB)

During my time of traveling throughout the United States for work, I carried a devotional book called *Thirty-One Days of Praise* by Ruth Myers. Each day I would read the devotion for that day and write notes in the margins regarding the challenges of my work life. I read that book every month for several years. I was beginning the path of spiritual healing and that started with praise for all that had occurred.

> Day 11 — I'm so grateful that all my past circumstances were permitted by You to make me see my need of You and prepare my heart for Your word. You draw me to Yourself, and to work out Your good purposes for my life.

I found information on the Internet about breast implant illness. Visiting two different plastic surgeons, meeting with the nurses and the surgery director required me to have good questions and believe in the direction I should go.

> "I will instruct you and teach you in the way which you should go; I will counsel you with My eye upon you." Psalm 32:8 (NASB)

"Who needs to hear your story of survival?" is written beside these verses in my Bible.

> "For the Spirit God gave us does not make us timid, but gives us power, love and self-discipline." 2 Timothy 1:7 (NIV)

> "And now I entrust you to God and the message of his grace that is able to build you up and give you an inheritance with all those he has set apart for himself." Acts 20:32 (NLT)

I believe God allows things into our life for a reason. No experience is wasted. He wants us to comfort others through the power He gave us to survive. It was not by my own strength, and even though I do not like telling my stories, they may be helpful for someone else.

A fire hose is used to put out fires. It is so strong and powerful it sometimes takes more than one person to hold it. It is connected to a pressurized hydrant or to a truck filled with water. If you need a fire hose, then something is on fire. In my story of breast cancers and breast implant illness, I hold the fire hose with God.

Over thirty years later, I think about my "fire hose" stories, and I know there is only one way I survived. God. I am an avid Bible reader. I pray, read scripture, rest, fight, and do it again. I am saved by the love of God.

"When you pass through the waters, I will be with you; And through the rivers, they will not overflow you. When you walk through the fire, you will not be scorched, Nor will the flame burn you. For I am the LORD your God, The Holy One of Israel, your Savior." Isaiah 43:2–3a (NASB)

Death has been a constant part of my adult life. I know it is coming someday, and the hard times have felt like I was being punished sometimes. But I am alive and thriving and therefore, you too can continue living well, if just for today.

"I will not die, but live, And tell of the works of the LORD. The LORD has disciplined me severely, but He has not given me over to death." Psalm 118:17–18 (NASB)

Do you believe that God wants a connection with you? The Bible tells us God, the Creator, loves us. Yet as sinners, we are separated from the holy God and cannot have a connection with Him.

God sent His only Son to take the punishment for our sins. He, as a perfect man, gave His life taking your sins to the cross. He took your place. He made a connection with God possible.

The Bible says, "If you confess with your mouth Jesus as Lord, and believe in your heart that God raised Him from the dead, you will be saved" (Romans 10:9 NASB). If you have never made a decision to follow Christ as your Savior, and if you would like to have the changed and eternal life God promised, pray silently in your own mind or say aloud the following words.

I believe Jesus is God's Son and is the only way to heaven. I believe He died for me to pay the penalty for my sin, rose from the dead, and lives today in heaven. I invite You, Jesus, to come for me, for my entire story and all my messes, and I want to make You Lord of my life. I want to submit all my choices to You. Thank You, Jesus, for the gift of eternal life that begins today. Thank You, Jesus, that You forgive my sins, and want to restore a close relationship between God and me.

Chapter 8

Marriage and Facebook
Saved My Life

I have perused my journals for the next ten years and find no constant illness. There is no record of migraines, herpes outbreaks, or diarrhea. The stress from work was hard, and my career was my focus for the next decade. I advanced in my jobs with different healthcare companies and traveled from Colorado throughout the West as a regional marketing director.

I relocated to Chicago for another company from 2005 to 2007. I was in charge of the marketing for twenty hospitals from Kansas City, Kansas, to Pittsburgh, Pennsylvania, and traveled constantly. During that time, I saw a chiropractor regularly, spoke of being tired, but the symptoms that had plagued me from 1996-2002 are not mentioned in my journals.

Realistically, I believed I had recovered from chemotherapy and radiation and was well. I now think I also was detoxing from the silicone that had leaked from the ruptured implant. No one had told me I would be sick for years or that silicone could create havoc with my immune system.

During 2007, I had to have my ovaries removed. I had decided to have genetic testing done by the University of Chicago. The genetic abnormality results showed I had a fifty percent chance of having ovarian cancer by the time I was fifty. I turned fifty in 2007, so I had them removed.

The return to Colorado Springs was challenging with periods of unemployment, but less stress. I found jobs that paid me much less and were below my skill set, but I could be at home at night. After being on the road up to 10,000 air miles per month for eight years, it was a blessing.

I did not have documented symptoms of illness related to my breast implant for ten years until 2012. The job stress was less, and I started a new phase of my career in senior healthcare. It started with a dog. Maybe. I know now it did not rupture the second implant, but I was really hurt from a friend's dog jumping on me and me falling to the ground. Hard. On my back. There is an increased level of discomfort and illness that begins after ten years of relative health.

Journal

June 9, 2012

The crazy brown Labrador goes home tomorrow. After he jumped on me and knocked me on my back six days ago, it has been a week of healing. Bruised, neck, back, and a three-inch bloody scratch. I could not exercise because of the pain. I had a massage yesterday and my right arm was so weak, I could not lift it. The swelling has decreased.

July 5, 2012

Pain lingers at a three or four. My lower back popped and the middle thoracic still has intense pain. My shoulders slump to escape the pain. Essential oils help, but I knock myself out with Excedrin PM nightly to sleep.

July 6, 2012

I said no to keeping another dog and must stop walking another friend's dogs. I have had eight days of pain and finally my shoulder popped into place this morning and the pain eased. What if it was never-ending?

July 8, 2012

Loneliness. Give up. I wish I had NOT lived after breast cancer fifteen years ago. Darkness and suicidal thoughts hit me like a brick. It has been such a struggle to survive. I cannot find the blessings today. Where is the hope?

July 13, 2012

I woke up happy. No pain, just twinges in my neck. I have not exercised for over two weeks and have to start over. I had massive diarrhea yesterday morning. It was uncontrollable. I stopped by the side of the road and cannot stop it. Nerves, digestion, and infectious disease must be cleansed using essential oils. If I did not use these things I would have been to the doctor and chiropractor. Twelve solid days of pain, but I am better now.

September 12, 2012

They put on a new roof at work and my head turned foggy from the fumes.

September 17, 2012

I feel God is protecting and preparing me for something, and I am ready and open to change. I must start looking for another job.

November 13, 2012

Three people I know died of cancer this week. All of them were young, some younger than me. The new job is allowing me to get the roof replaced and other repairs from hail damage in the summer. I have survived a five-year "desert" of money followed by the summer's deadly wildfires and a fall of transition.

December 20, 2012

I have been praying for a deeper relationship, friendships and even male friendships to test and prove I could trust again. I also prayed not to spend Christmas alone. My Bible study leaders were invited to a party at a male leader's house to celebrate his late wife's life and her love of Christmas. She had died in July after more than two years fighting cancer.

At the party, the leader asked me to join him and his kids for Christmas. It would be their first Christmas without their wife and mother and grandmother, so I said I would think about it. I had told God I would say yes to the first invitation, but it was so unexpected. He had decorated the house with six Christmas trees.

I have always said God would have to put someone in my life and say, 'Walk here and go there,' for me to even be approachable. I have been happily divorced and alone for almost ten years. I have spent time healing emotionally and physically and learning more about God.

January 7, 2013

I am up at 4:30 a.m. with shoulder pain. Even though I had help to move the Christmas boxes downstairs, I hurt so badly.

January 22, 2013

My shoulder is fine; it is in my neck that I have problems. I have to have an MRI next and look for degenerative disc disease.

February 5, 2013

Bulging disc in my neck at C6, C7, and T1 or in my cervical spine and thoracic spine, and it is worse on my left side as seen in an MRI. A bone spur is irritating the cervical nerve, and it looks like it is pushing out 1/8 inch. I crashed. I felt sadness, more pain, anticipating disability and limitation and damage. Next week I will begin physical therapy and traction. I become disoriented, hearing in my mind, "You will be a cripple with degenerating disc disease." I changed my pillow to a flat one and have to do neck stretches adding essential oils to help with the pain.

February 7, 2013

I went back to the gym today but NO upper back or neck weights. I can walk and use free weights on my lower body only.

February 25, 2013

The tooth abscess explains the face as I waited five more days to seek help. I was pretty sick. The following week I had food poisoning possibly on Wednesday night and was throwing up and had diarrhea. I have lost four pounds in two weeks. The infection was awful and I cannot take any antibiotics.

March 25, 2013

I had a rough night in the emergency room with kidney stones and the most incredible pain of my life. At 1:00 a.m. I called a friend to take me to the ER. I was throwing up and writhing in pain until the morphine kicked in finally.

March 27, 2013

No more oncologist appointments after twenty-six years and fifteen years. My doctor said, "You are done, a cancer survivor, and I do not want to see you again except socially!" Almost one half of my life I have gone to an oncologist regularly. (He emphatically told me that I did not need to have my implant removed and replaced. The risk of surgery was greater than the implant. How wrong he was!) Kidney stones, neck pain, and infection, but I am happy and in love.

April 8, 2013

Allergies? No sleep. Another migraine, red sore stuffy nose is miserable.

May 9, 2013

I awoke with pain in the neck and numbness in my right hand.

Throughout the spring of 2013, Ed and I continued to explore a romantic relationship. From meeting at the Christmas party, through counseling, long talks and much prayer, we decided to proceed in a relationship which led to marriage. He knew my cancer history, and I knew he was able to cope with my illnesses. We followed the path God put us both on, which was to love one another and trust in future happiness.

May 19, 2013

Ed and I became engaged and are to be married on October 5, 2013.

The thrill of love dominates my journals for months. After our marriage in October, we went to Hawaii for two weeks for our honeymoon. I cannot believe this wonderful man chose me to be his life partner. Happiness followed us everywhere we went: Road to Hana, swimming with turtles and dolphins, ocean kayaking, and snorkeling in the crystal waters of Oahu and Maui. Life is turning into a fantasy of love.

I did not record much of my physical challenges in my journals as I was focused on my new marriage and my spiritual life. I do remember recurrent sores in my vaginal and labia area were very painful. The dryness in my female parts sent me to the physician for prescribed estrogen creams.

I had anxiety with all the changes in my life. A new consulting job working part-time for a healthcare company started after a few months. We had decided to move into my home so I was emptying out his house, painting, stripping wallpaper, and deep cleaning the three-story house. We decided to rent the house in the spring of 2014.

My parents made a decision to move to Colorado in August 2014, and the preparation for their arrival was a time of joy and stress. It was the first time in my adult life that I did not work full-time.

We traveled to Europe for three weeks in October 2014 and enjoyed the lack of home responsibilities. When we returned, we had the experience of holidays with all the blended family. It was a good time and I was relatively healthy. My food sensitivities were increasing, and I could no longer eat hummus or anything with chickpeas. I was using my herpes medicine daily to keep the sores away and started to need anti-anxiety medication more frequently.

Journal

2014

January 7, 2014

The numbness in my hands is so bad again, both right and left hands. The right thumb was so numb that I could not play the piano well. Prayer, oils, traction, massage, and ice, and I was better.

February 5, 2014

We cannot have sex as my back pain takes over. Pain for me is down to 4–5, and I can get in and out of bed and chair without crying out in pain. The week has been a blur with pain. Simple things: sit, walk, stand, and yet they take all my energy.

It has been three years since I have had this kind of back pain. God saying, "Enough, slow down, rest."

February 24, 2014

This is my first day with no illness and no back problem in a month.

May 29, 2014

My back is better after seeing the chiropractor and treating with essential oils. No sharp pain, only a dull ache. My throat is dry and sore from talking too much.

June 2, 2014

Skin cancer on my nose, not a bad one, but another cancer. It looks bad, and they have to take more of the nose out. I had a massage last week and it helped my back and neck. Surgery is scheduled for 6/12/2014.

June 14–24, 2014

We traveled to Seattle, Portland, Oregon (where I had my nose stitches out), Northern California, and Napa Valley for my cousin's wedding. I had a case of hives from the antibiotics after surgery. Then we flew to Indiana for my aunt and uncle's fiftieth wedding anniversary. Crazy schedule.

June 29, 2014

Went to a follow-up with my plastic surgeon. He was not satisfied with his work on my nose and wanted to do another surgery. Maybe later.

We planned to open an escape room business in May 2015 and were consumed with design, construction, equipment, website, and processes that took most of my time for the first four months. I was teaching healthcare management at the University of Phoenix in the evenings throughout this time. I was busy and not well. Again.

Journal

January 1, 2015

Depression is beginning. I am not ready for the escape rooms to open for our escape room business. The students do not feel I make time for them. Do I have cancer again? I am not spending enough time with my parents after they moved here. I have had no income for seven months and need to have my own money. We decided to paint our entire house and do minor construction projects. I have no memory of the holidays, no music, no relaxation. I was just working.

January 2, 2015

Why depression? Pain? Sadness? Holiday blues? My husband's daughter's families were struggling. Two grandsons have gone to live with their fathers. I say no to food, sugar, and alcohol for now.

February 3, 2015

What do I need to recover from? Fear of failure? What is not working for me in my life?

Lord of Creation,
Create in us a new rhythm of life
Composed of hours that sustain
Rather than stress,
Of days that deliver
Rather than destroy.
Of time that tickles
Rather than tackles.

Common Prayer: A Liturgy for Ordinary Radicals[7]

February 10, 2015

I have gone through a deep time of spiritual healing through numerous pathways. Prayer, meditation, Sozo healing, and solitude are part of my life. Healing is hard work, but I want to understand why I am always sick. How much is physical? How much of my illness is spiritual?

Yesterday, I had a bowel movement while driving. It is so awful, dirty, shameful, and disgusting to have uncontrollable bowels. My desire is for health and productivity.

February 27, 2015

I have had a herpes outbreak for the last two days. Herpes has hampered my normalcy and increased my pain. We have had snow for three days and I have not left the house.

March 11, 2015

Headache. Migraine. Sick. Nausea. Pray against illness and evil in my life. The brain fog is gone, and the pain and nausea are gone. My neck is sore from too much caffeine. When did I "beat myself up" to keep going and then take a break, I lie down and "beat myself up" again for pausing.

April 1, 2015

Lay down your burden of having to live at a breathless pace. I remain tired and nauseous most of the time and it is scary. I have been drinking too much alcohol, which is not good.

April 7, 2015

My neck is hurting after cleaning the whole house and vacuuming is so hard to do. Allergies are bad, so I used the massage machine for thirty minutes. I need to sleep, but my congestion is severe.

May 19, 2015

We are both sick with the flu or a cold or allergies. I have been so sick that I cried. Alcohol rinse, cough drops, cough expectorant, and aches, and nothing helps. When I woke up, I could not breathe as I was hacking with lots of phlegm. Lord, help me to recover.

May 25, 2015

Finally, I awoke after seven hours of sleep and feel better and can breathe. My foot is hurting with pain like plantar fasciitis and swelling. I had to go to acute care, use a cane, and take some pain medicine.

I have missed a whole week of work to illness. I think I have a quarter size hole of water bronchitis stuck in my lungs. Opening a business and preparing his house for selling may be too much.

July 14, 2015

I was sick with painful bladder pain and pain on urination. I cannot hold my urine now. Between my husband's hip replacement surgery in early July, running a business, trying to sell his house, and a granddaughter in the hospital for mental health problems, I have to keep going during a tough time.

July 24, 2015

My husband is feeling better after being hospitalized for multiple pulmonary blood clots, twenty small ones, and one big clot. It was a side effect of his hip replacement surgery. He has to be on oxygen for twenty days and on a blood thinner for six months.

I hate July because everything bad in my life happens in July. My neck went out Friday, but I am better today. The granddaughter is out of the hospital, my husband is recovering, the house sold, and I can handle the amount of business so far.

July 30, 2015

His daughter is in jail and may serve time now. So sad. There were outstanding warrants for her and the rehabilitation place in Denver turned her in. That is all we know. We will not pay her bond because we think she used rehabilitation in the past to hide from the consequences of her actions.

August 15, 2015

Do I have nose cancer again? It has been a hard week for my husband who went back to work full time, the car is in the shop, grandsons that have been taken and placed with their fathers, and a daughter who demands money while in jail. I am still waiting to hear about the biopsy on my nose and will wait and watch.

September 8, 2015

We were busy getting the third room open for our escape room business all week. I ended with a migraine at church. I took my migraine medicine and slept for thirteen hours. We have two busy weeks ahead of us.

2016

February 2, 2016

We went to New York to see his mother in January, and I had to recover from vacation for three days. My neck is healed with all the walking we did in New York City and less stress. I have fought depression and had an anxiety attack when I returned.

Snow is starting again with blowing. We have a warm furnace and I have a warm and loving husband. My shoulder hurts and my hands are numb when I play the piano.

The busyness of life overwhelmed my schedule and the summer and fall had been too much for me to pay attention to my own health. Always increasing illnesses, husband and his family issues, and operating a business for a few months had taken its toll. I was constantly sick with something. Head cold. Herpes. Pain in the neck area. Back issues. Breathing issues. I was using essential oils to keep going.

One night, I could not sleep. Sitting on the couch in the middle of the night, struggling to breathe, and I found a Facebook post on something called breast implant illness. BII. What is that?

Reading the list of symptoms of breast implant illness, I understood.

I finally knew what was wrong with me. I had had the second saline implant since 1998, eighteen years ago. The light bulb went on. I had so many of the symptoms and yet, no doctor had been able to find out anything definitively wrong with me. Doctors said, "It is age. It is early menopause. It is stress."

As I touched the implant, I realized it was hard. Sometimes it was pliable and sometimes I could not lie on my stomach comfortably because of the grapefruit in my chest. Reading the symptoms list was surreal, and I had clear recognition of my own breast implant illness. I was shaking, sick to my stomach, angry, and relieved. Now what do I do about the replaced saline eighteen-year-old implant for reconstruction following my second breast cancer that is making me sick.

I joined a few Facebook groups centered on BII and scrolled through the comments of women who had illnesses as I had and some who were very sick. There were thousands of women on these sites and social media was exploding with women helping other women.

One Facebook site, Breast Implant Illness Warriors, stated "We are here to help support you from the moment you thought it, help you get through the next step, help you get explanted by recommended surgeons who do the proper explant technique and suggestions on what helped us to heal. Many opinions are here but the focus is love and help. ..." It now has over 8,000 members as of 2020.

The lists of symptoms are different on various sites, but I remember consistencies between lists from different sources. My list of symptoms included: fatigue, brain fog, memory loss, joint pain, poor sleep, dry eyes and blurry vision, cough, gastrointestinal issues (many allergies to food), persistent viral infections, ear ringing, headaches, ocular migraines, weight problems, heart palpitations, sore and aching joints especially shoulders, feet, and back, skin rashes, low libido, frequent urination, anxiety, depression and panic attacks, feeling like I was dying, and bowel and bladder problems.

I had had a complete heart work up a couple of years before this in 2014 for a racing heartbeat at over 150 beats per minute during a hike. Hiking up a mountain as I usually did each weekend, my heart rate went high on a fairly level path. I thought I was having a heart attack. After sitting for several minutes my heart rate decreased to 136. I started wearing a Fitbit to monitor my heart rate and keep it below 140. Every heart test was normal: lab work, echocardiogram, EKG, and stress test.

I had had a thyroid biopsy in 2011, as my thyroid was palpable. It was negative for cancer. When I exercised, I hurt everywhere. If I didn't exercise, the pain in my joints was worse. I continued three times a week with weight training, walking, and hiking.

I had a constant skin rash on my neck area when I used essential oils even if they were diluted. Lavender and frankincense were especially toxic to my skin. Now I believe it was drawing out the toxins in some way. I had no underarm hair at all. The sores and tenderness in my vaginal and labia area were awful for a new bride.

The worst symptom for me was the loss of bowel and bladder control. This had developed over a period of four years. I knew where every bathroom was around the city and even where parks were with large bushes. I will not describe the accidents that were beyond embarrassing. This culminated in me carrying underwear in my car. I had no control over my bodily functions, but I was only 54, and did not want to wear adult diapers!

Comments from women on the Facebook sites echoed experiences like mine: "I have experienced almost all of them." "I have had a few of them." "I tested positive for this." "I tested negative for this." "I had so many of these." "I think I am dying."

There were many symptoms I did not have: hair loss, dry skin, thyroid issues, easy bruising, leaky gut, acid reflux, pancreatitis, chronic fatigue, night sweats, fungal or candida infections. I was never diagnosed with all the different autoimmune diseases listed: fibromyalgia, Lyme, EBV Raynaud's Syndrome, rheumatoid arthritis, scleroderma, lupus, multiple sclerosis, or Sjogren's Syndrome.

From various sources on the web, there are many other symptoms listed, such as fatigue, chest pain, hair loss, body odor, chills, photosensitivity, chronic pain, neurological and hormonal issues. Lists of implant complications include: implant rupture, bruising, bleeding, skin necrosis, scar tissue buildup (capsular contracture), implant deflation, change in breast shape, change in the volume of the implant, or sensation, nipple discharge, asymmetry, and need for further surgery.

Even Google and Pinterest have pages of symptoms of BII which included all the above symptoms as well as disorientation, vertigo, premature aging, dry mouth, sinus congestion, constant need to clear throat, temperature intolerance, sensitivity to light or sound, slow healing, swollen or tender lymph nodes, inflammation, weight gain, hysterectomy, dehydration, liver, kidney and gallbladder problems, leaky gut, irritable bowel syndrome, pins and needles, painful ribs and circulation issues.

Are there any tests that indicate a connection between breast implants and symptoms that are being labelled Breast Implant Illness (BII)?

"There is no diagnostic test specifically for Breast Implant Illness (BII). This is one of the current areas of focus for the Aesthetic Surgery Education and Research Foundation (ASERF), the research arm of The Aesthetic Society. There are, however, tests for autoimmune diseases. Some patients who report having Breast Implant Illness (BII) have positive tests and others have negative tests for autoimmune diseases."[8]

No wonder the medical establishment is confused and unaware of a specific illness. The symptoms were as varied as the women who visited their doctors and were referred to multiple specialists. I realized there were no tests to confirm my suspicion, so I did not go to my primary care physician regarding this potential diagnosis.

Chapter 9

Explant and Results

Facebook Post 3/11/2016

I had my first breast cancer at thirty and second cancer at forty-one on the other side. I had silicone way back in 1987, and it ruptured after being thrown from my horse. At forty, I remember saying "if I am always going to feel this way I don't want to live."

I MADE THEM TAKE THE IMPLANT OUT AND EXCHANGE IT in 1998 during the lumpectomy on the other breast.

The surgeon did say the first implant was ruptured and even though it was exchanged for a saline one, he didn't believe it caused the pain and sickness of my second cancer.

Now after eighteen years without cancer of the breasts, I am tired of pain, constant gut problems, allergies, immune system issues, etc. I had decided it was chemo reactions, age, and illness.

Then I read your story and have 60 percent of the symptoms of BII. I have made appointments to get tests and get this implant removed. At the worst, I will no longer have it in me and be a bit poorer; at the best I can live the rest of my life healthier. Thanks so much!

My search began for plastic surgeons that would consult and remove my implant in my geographical area of Colorado. Because I have a medical background, I made a list of the qualifications I wanted in a physician, questions to ask, and did not use any "approved" physician from any lists on Facebook.

The next step was to find a doctor and get the toxic bag out of me. I read Facebook pages and searched the Internet for what I needed in a plastic surgeon. I also had to begin to figure out how to pay for an explant.

Within a week from the revelation, I had a list of questions for a physician and three physicians I wanted to visit for appointments. I wanted to have a documented evaluation of the inflammation in my body before and after surgery. I found a laboratory that would take my implant and evaluate the actual physical structure and the liquid inside it for anything that was not saline. There was a lot to accomplish in a short time frame.

First, I scheduled an appointment with a nurse practitioner who did thermography breast imaging. Thermography is a physiologic test that demonstrates thermal patterns in skin temperature that may be normal or which may indicate disease or other abnormality. It is a controversial alternative medical test that is not covered by insurance. You stand before a sensitive heat-imaging machine and get a colored picture of heat being expended by your body. These were some results before the removal of my saline implant on my right side.

Head and neck: Some diffuse increase is present at the anterolateral (front/side) neck and appears to be lymph related.

Breast: Hyperthermia at the right breast may correspond to an inflammatory process involving the implant or the overlying soft tissues. The left breast is noted to be cool overall.

Back: Increase of heat at the central upper back more so towards the left is indicative of increased muscular tension. Accentuation of the upper thoracic levels is indicative of underlying joint inflammation.

Abdomen: Specific intensity immediately subjacent to the left breast (no implant) appears related to costochondral inflammation.

Upper Extremities: Some specific heat intensity is evident towards the right brachial plexus. The hands are warm bilaterally and a pre-diabetic condition may have relevance.

Discussion: The thermal findings in the reconstructed right breast should be considered to be at some risk for developing pathology or breast disease.

What I saw in the pictures made me concerned and relieved. I was concerned that my neck, chest, breast, and lymph nodes where the implant was, were colorful in a heated red. The left side, no implant side, was blue-green. My upper back was red, orange, and yellow and corresponded to pain in my body. What does this mean? I wasn't sure, but my body was telling me something.

I reviewed many plastic surgeons' websites and their reviews, both out of my geographical areas and even out of the country. There were "approved" lists of physicians on the Facebook pages with videos and philosophy of practice. I looked for doctors with good clinical training and a length of time in practice. Most, if not all, the plastic surgeons also insert breast implants for breast reconstruction or for cosmetic augmentation (make the breasts larger) as part of their medical practice. People on the Facebook pages chose doctors because of recommendations of other patients and from these "approved lists."

What criteria did people use to select an approved plastic surgeon?

- Do they believe in breast implant illness?
- Will they listen to me and take time with me?
- Do they have experience in en bloc capsulectomy as a procedure?
- How much do they charge and what is the total cost?
- How long will I have to wait for consults and surgery?
- Do they take my insurance or are they in-network with their insurance?
- Are they on an approved "list"? How credible is this list?
- Are they close to where I live?
- Must be willing to remove the entire capsule around implant.
- What are their recommendations about replacing the implant?
- What is my comfort level with the staff and doctor?
- If I choose to travel to a doctor, what services do they provide pre- and post-surgery, as it is an outpatient procedure? For example: Nurses visit post-surgery, transportation to and from hotel and office, follow-up care and hotels recommended?

There was much discussion on the Internet regarding payment for explant. Would insurance pay for it? How much did it cost? Why did the implant manufacturing companies not pay for the damage caused and pay to have an explant? Some women were so ill and not able to work, and now they are trying to navigate the payment of their explant with help from social media, phone calls, and emails.

There were questions about what "medical codes" the physician had to use in order to determine if the insurance paid for the procedure. What codes caused the explant to be excluded from coverage from insurance.

There are online videos showing how to get your insurance to pay some, if not all, of the cost of explant.

It seemed as if the best chance of being covered by insurance was diagnosis of capsular contraction, pain, or previous breast cancer. The cost seemed to range widely from $8,000 to $17,000 depending on the location, procedure, and the correction to the remaining breast or tissue that was required.

Family, spouses, kids, friends, and co-workers were the next obstacle to manage, according to Facebook. My husband was very supportive as were my parents. They listened to me and had watched my health decline for years. Other breast cancer friends were sympathetic and wondered if they faced the same issue with their implants after their breast cancer. Strangers were telling me they had cosmetic implants and no one knew, and they asked me to keep them informed on the process.

Other patients with breast implant illness did not have the same positive reactions. Some spouses enjoyed the bigger breasts and did not want any changes. Some did not want their spouse or girlfriend to have an elective, potentially risky surgery when there was no proof the implant was the cause of the illnesses. Getting their families to resources like books and TV shows helped them see it was not simply a group of women on Facebook who were sick and hysterical.

The most challenging group to convince of the reality of breast implant illness is the medical establishment. Physicians would recommend being healthier by exercise, physical therapy, and stop smoking and drinking to any and all of our vague symptoms. The women would try different medications and their primary care physician would refer people to multiple specialists including: rheumatology, cardiology, neurology, infectious disease, and psychiatry.

I finally went to my primary care doctor and gave him links to adverse reactions to implants. I showed him some research I had found on the effects of ruptured implants, long term issues with implants, and the list of symptoms. He helped me with referrals to plastic surgeons in my area. He became supportive after the explant when he saw the change in my health and the positive changes in my blood results and weight.

My search for a qualified explant plastic surgeon identified three physicians, two an hour away in Denver, and one in Colorado Springs where I lived. I scheduled an appointment in Denver, but the other doctor in Denver had a wait time for explant of four months. The office in Denver was very fancy and had pictures of famous people that had been their patients. It was intimidating, but the staff was friendly as they took my history and were interested in my story. The doctor was not surprised by my request, had had recent training in en bloc capsulectomy, and I left hopeful.

My next visit was to a plastic surgeon in Colorado Springs where I lived. I had my list of questions, and he was honest and forthright. He did not believe that implants could cause all of my symptoms, but he had no other explanation for my illnesses. He was an older physician and had done hundreds of total capsule

emovals with explant in the late 1980s when he was a resident training in plastic
urgery in North Carolina.

At that time, silicone implants were being removed regularly as a result of
eing pulled off the market. This was at the same time I was living overseas and
vas never notified of potential risks of silicone implants. I had even been on TV as
young cancer patient, very satisfied with her silicone implant and her decision.
ven though he did not believe in BII, he would remove them.

We discussed whether I was going to have any reconstruction with another
mplant, a lift taken from my stomach fat and muscles, or going flat. I had seen
ictures and had investigated these three possibilities as well as other things. I
ecided to be flat with prosthesis.

There are so many options; it can become overwhelming to decide what you
vant and what your body can tolerate. Recovery time, risks, potential outcomes,
urrent health, cost and personal preferences are all things to consider for the
xplant procedure and any reconstruction.

The plastic surgeon's nurse let me know she did not believe in BII of any kind,
nd I was one of only a few people who had ever wanted an explant.

That was sad for me, but think of her position. Who would knowingly do
omething harmful to people day after day and be in the healing profession? She
aid all of my symptoms are consistent with aging, post-menopausal, and cancer
istory with chemotherapy. I ignored the negativity.

I met with the plastic surgeon's business office manager to discuss costs,
nsurance, and scheduling the procedure. She informed me that as a breast cancer
urvivor the insurance I had (Tricare), had to pay for any post-mastectomy
rocedures by federal law. I would have some expense, but not overwhelming.
hat is not the case for cosmetic surgery patients as it is considered completely
n elective surgery. If the patient does not have documented pain and or scarred
ontraction of the capsule around the implant, most insurance will refuse to
ay for the procedure. Even if the women are desperately sick, if there is not a
efinitive medical link showing causation between breast implants and a myriad of
utoimmune and vague symptoms, insurance will not cover the explant procedure
et.

The next step was assuring myself that the doctor would take pictures of the
mplants, save them for me, and direct the pathology laboratory not to destroy the
mplants, as I wanted to send them to a lab for testing. This required a meeting with
he director of nursing at the ambulatory surgery center he used. The director of
ursing was agreeable and would make sure the proper requests were made to the

pathology department at the hospital. The implants had to go there for testing for cancer, and that would take a week after my surgery.

I would follow-up with the laboratory and pathologist to pick up my implants when they were finished with them.

The next statement the director of nursing said surprised me. "I have breast implants, my second set, and I have wondered whether they are making me sick." The surgery center did hundreds of breasts implants every year, both for reconstruction and for cosmetic purposes. She was very interested and asked me to return in a month and tell her how my health had changed or if it did not. (I did return to see her and give her my good news of improving health after removal of my implant.)

Surgery was scheduled for the following week. My parents and my husband came with me to surgery and prayed for my safety. The doctor had brought his own camera to take pictures, but took my husband's camera, so we would have an immediate record of the implant after explant.

I went home to recover for a few days and rested. The drain that was inserted in the surgery area was the most painful thing of the whole procedure. I went back to the plastic surgeon's office at one week for the drain to be removed. I saw the physician briefly and the nurse took out the drain. Whoosh! OUCH!

Even though I was seeing an overall improvement in my health and decrease of symptoms, it felt like they believed I was psychosomatic. In other words, I felt better, because I wanted and needed to feel better. I returned for my follow-up visit two weeks after surgery. The only thing the physician and his nurse could not understand was my complete restoration of bowel and bladder control. In two weeks. Every other symptom could be age, menopause, and post-chemotherapy, but not bowel and bladder control. They were happy because I was elated.

Throughout the next three months, my skin and eyes became brighter and changed noticeably to others. The neck rashes disappeared. Aching of my joints became minimal, and I was not hurting after mild exercise or taking a walk. My vision had cleared and my eyes were no longer dry. The brain fog and memory loss lessened even after anesthesia for the surgery.

I still could not eat dairy or wheat, but my chronic diarrhea had abated. No migraines, panic attacks, or heart palpitations in the two weeks following the surgery. I had no herpes breakout or any cold symptoms. I was still coughing and my ears still were ringing. The anxiety, irritability, and depression decreased and my whole being seemed "lighter." Best of all, I no longer felt I was slowly dying.

Healing may not occur immediately. I had experienced years with a defective aline implant, years with a ruptured silicone implant, and many years of illness. I needed to be patient with myself as I recovered.

Confirmation of my defective implant came from Innoval Laboratories in Ottawa, Canada, which was a recommended lab for testing of the implant. In 2016, the cost for analysis of my implant was $500 and the wait time for results was six months. They took my implant because they had not had anyone from Colorado correspond with them. I received a Failure Analysis Report seven months after I sent them my implant. I had included all my physician notes from both implants and the post-surgical picture my physician took with the implant.

My implant was a Mentor style 1600 saline inflatable sold under Catalog Number 350-1645. I had this information from my surgical notes from eighteen years previous. Its manufacturing attributes correlated with products made in the nineties1990s. My report read as follows:

"The implant was defectively made from the outset, however, the shell is neither perforated or ruptured. The filling valve components are defective and mismatched. The condition of the shell establishes that the implant passed through cycles of over-inflation and under-inflation during its dwell time, a consequence of an incompetent valving system. The filling fluid is grossly contaminated with evidence of microbiological activity."

I was relieved, shocked, and sad for myself and every other woman with similar implants in their bodies. Trusting the doctors, hospitals, and manufacturer of the implant had left me feeling betrayed.

I sent an email to Dr. P. Blais, Ph.D. F.C.I.C. in October 2016 after my explant in May 2016, outlining my concern about the possible long-term respiratory and cardiac impacts of the implant following an episode I had while hiking that fall. Dr. Blais responded,

"With reference to your email of October 28, 2016, and the statement regarding cardiac issues, I offer the following. Cardiac function is frequently affected by breast implants. The effect can be strictly mechanical and related to the constant pressure an implant and its capsule exert on the chest. Thus, cardiac-like symptoms would be encountered. However, it is unlikely that this process would affect the heart rate. A second pathway can be a side effect of pharmaceutical treatments or alterations in serologic parameters.

Other influential factors could be respiratory. Implants impact drastically on respiratory function. Long-term implant users are more severely affected and the mechanism relates to alterations in intercostal muscle atrophy or chest wall damage. According to this view, an impaired breathing function could initiate cardiac-like symptoms and alterations in cardiac rate. For my part, I would favor a wait-and-see approach in combination with a conscious effort to rehabilitate breathing habits."

He took the time to explain what happened to my first silicone implant according to the surgeon's notes, which I provided to him. The Surgitek, Dow Corning implant had two shells or double lumens. These implants were unreliable and lost the outer shell contents within a few years. They also were subject to severe contamination of this outer compartment through the backflow of body fluids and microorganisms. Add to the manufacturing defect, the fall from the horse and the subsequent rupture of the implant led to my first round of BII, I am sure.

The second implant was puckered, demonstrating that at one time, it held more fluid than when it was extracted. There were two "puckers," which showed collateral erosion and disruption of the shell and demonstrated that, at one time, the implant fluid had been below the optimum recommended amount. The laboratory showed that the valve used to fill the implant was faulty and the cap did not stay on when it was out of the body. The valve leaked fluid visibly upon pressure. That explained why sometimes my implant would be hard and sometimes soft, but I was never informed to look for this condition as a potentially harmful problem.

I had requested an en bloc or full capsule removal and it was performed by my plastic surgeon. The Innoval laboratory also examined the capsule. Where the valve had been inside my body, there was a cluster of bloody tissue, which suggested to them, infiltration of blood into the implant. The valve cap was also entangled with capsular tissue. The pathologist reported the capsule tissue as dense fibrosis and foreign body giant cell reaction. Yikes!

Upon examination of the implant, the laboratory reached the following conclusion: "Cycles of inflation and deflation (of the implant) could have been many during a span of 18 years, but the outcome would have been the same, culminating in the exchange of the original saline solution for protein-laden body fluids with the occasional adventitious inoculate of viable micro-organisms."

My conclusion: My implant was contaminated with microorganisms, which grew and then were expelled back into my body through a faulty valve. This caused a constant low-grade infection and ongoing inflammation for many years.

My body would have filled the implant through inflating it with body fluids and microorganisms until the implant was full and then it would empty out, exchanging these same contaminants over and over. When it emptied too much, the implant changed shape. It could have easily completely ruptured, expelling this contaminated fluid throughout my chest.

"Examination of the solution in the implant through trans illumination revealed urbidity consistent with spores and fine microbiological debris. Visible aggregates of white microbiological material were also noted and the debris had a clearly ibrillar flocculent character. Magnified examination through the shell confirmed nycobacterial entities. In addition, biofilm adhered to the inside surface of the shell, confirming that some of the microbiological activity was in the form of cooperative colonies partly bound to the elastomer surface," according to the Innoval report.

Further, the Innoval report stated: "The implant was subject to microbiological contamination and exposed her to long term low-grade infective processes. Alterations in her immunochemical profile would be expected to remain, at least for some time. These observations suggest that the implant site had an 'abscess-like' character of longstanding origin."

In my words: The inside of the implant showed mold spores and a slimy surface of bacteria adhering to the inside of the implant. The valve was an abscess, a boil, angry and untreated for years. The implant was exchanging contaminated bacteria-filled fluids into and out of my body. The implant was making me very sick.

Journal

September 29, 2016

I was sick with bowel and bladder problems for several hours with embarrassing stops in traffic jams. It is better and yet, I still have problems if I am not careful about what I eat.

October 1, 2016

Off to Mad Creek and Strawberry Fields Hot Springs trail in Steamboat Springs, Colorado, for 3.2 miles. It was scary difficult for me with a very high heart rate and stayed at 133 beats per min (BPM) for the entire trail. I also had chest and neck pain. After the hot springs, we headed back, and I led the way and BPM was at 119 or below. Six miles was a bit much, but we were in shape for it.

January 28, 2017

Boom. Phone rings. You have cancer on your nose. Basal cell this time and it is small but you will need surgery on February 8. Nausea. Stomach hurts. My mind shuts down. Anxiety and then peace.

God gave me Revelations 3:12 (NASB), "[S]he who overcomes, I will make a pillar in the temple of My God and [s]he will not go out from it anymore." I love life and have hope. I do not cry. One more challenge for this body, but this world is not my home.

February 16, 2017

One week and one day post-cancer surgery on my nose. I had an answered prayer; **I took an antibiotic without side effects. This has never happened since 1998, almost twenty years.**

I sent the following letter to my primary care doctor, plastic surgeon, and former oncologist. I felt I needed them to know what had happened to me and how BII felt to their former and current patient.

February 16, 2017

Dear Dr. T, Dr. H, and Dr. S:

Thank you for your care for me as primary care, plastic surgeon, and oncologist over the last 18 years. In May 2016, Dr. H. removed my right breast implant at my request. I was sick with many non-specific symptoms and am convinced I had breast implant illness.

The saline implant in the right breast was from 1998 when I had a lumpectomy in the left breast from breast cancer, and replaced the ruptured silicone implant in the right breast at the same time in Dallas. This was followed by chemotherapy and radiation in Colorado Springs. I was released from Dr. S.'s, my oncologist, care after 15 years in 2013.

Dr. T has been my primary care provider for twenty years and has worked with me on many of the non-specific symptoms I had. I had joint pain, inflammation, intestinal issues, severe allergies, mental fog, pain upon exercise and pain without exercise, racing heart rate, loss of bowel control, loss of bladder control, migraines, anxiety, exercise-induced asthma, and could not take any antibiotics without a reaction.

My symptoms started within 2 years after my second implant. The last antibiotic I took was Clindomycin in 2015 for a squamous cell carcinoma on my nose, and I broke out in hives.

Within 1 week of the en bloc capsulectomy by Dr. H. in May 2016, 70% of my symptoms were gone! I have had two migraines in nine months, and the joint pain is completely resolved, and I can even think clearly again. have had heart issues that have been evaluated, and even though they are still there (rapid heart rate), the cardiologist cannot find anything wrong with my heart.

Most importantly, I have control of my bowel and bladder functions again. I can finally drive to Denver without having to stop halfway at Monument and Castle Rock to go to the bathroom! A trip of one hour.

Two weeks ago, I had a basal cell carcinoma removed from my nose (February 2017 by Dr. C., dermatologist, and Dr. A., plastic surgeon). This is my fourth different cancer diagnosis. The amazing thing that happened is that Dr. A., plastic surgeon, prescribed Clindomycin again, and I had NO REACTION TO THE ANTIBIOTIC.

I have included a report on the removed implant and capsule done by a laboratory in Canada. As I suspected, the implant had mycobacteria and had a faulty valve, which resulted in body fluids being exchanged for a long time. I remember the implant becoming hard and then soft, but did not know why.

I share all this because you know my medical journey, and I want you to know the dangers that I unknowingly faced from the saline implant being in my body for 18 years. Obviously, not everyone has this reaction, but it is worth noting that if someone has many unexplained medical issues AND has a breast implant, there may be a connection.

Sincerely,

Debi

Journal

March 19, 2017

I am so humbled to make it to my sixty years old birthday and planning a trip to China.

Facebook Post 5/24/19

Three years, or 36 months ago in 2016, I explanted my breast implant (everyone in medicine thought implants were completely fine) after 18 years, multiple health issues, and finding a Facebook page about BII or breast implant illness. I thought I was dying at 59. I hiked, but had to stop often because of [sic] my heart rate went over 155 beats per minute. I finally sweat again now.

Yesterday, my husband and I hiked Red Rock Open Space in Colorado Springs, traipsed through a creek bed, climbed up boulders to get out of a canyon, and had an adventure. We are walking or climbing three to four miles per day.

Today: Hiked 4.7 miles, 660 feet elevation climb, 10,000 steps, and 120 heart rate or beats per minute. Get those toxic implants out of your life and LIVE!

Four years after explant, four cancers, and two rounds of breast implant illness have taken their toll. I expected to retire and hike in the Colorado mountains every day, but it is not to be. Many of us who have taken out our toxic implants identify as BII survivors and say, "The Heal is Real." I know for me, the journey through BII after being thrown from my horse was full of illness and there were times I thought I was dying. But I am alive, writing books, able to hike three times a week, exercise with weights, eat most things, and fully participate in life.

There is hope for you as well. You are not crazy. Women who have implants are fine. Women who have implants are sick. Women who have implants are thriving. Women who have implants are barely surviving. Which one of these women do you resemble? Sometime in your journey you may have identified with all of these situations.

May my journey to wholeness inspire you to make whatever changes you need to make: body, soul, spirit, and mind.

Chapter 10

Solutions for Wellness, Detoxification and Recovery

Detoxing was part of my life after my second breast cancer, chemotherapy, and radiation. I did not know that the silicone implant material that had ruptured and oozed into my body for nearly four years was also being removed through the detoxification. After I finished cancer treatment, I started a macrobiotic diet, which was popular in the 1990s.

When I discovered the negative effect on my digestive system with eating wheat and dairy, I have abstained to a great extent for twenty years. I do miss desserts, since most of them are made of either dairy and wheat or both. But the cramping, loose stools, and general inflammation that attack me for days after I have tiramisu, crème pie, or a doughnut are not worth it. Detoxification cleansing of the liver and colon at least four times a year following my second cancer, including my post-radiation coffee enemas, was my detoxification experience.

Nothing was going to keep my body healthy when I had a breast implant with a leaky valve that was allowing mold to grow in the implant and recycling toxic waste into my system. I had proof when I received the report detailing the examination of my explanted implant. But how can I improve my overall health and allow my body to heal itself? I turned to Abby Kurth, my friend and clinical nutritionist who had helped me survive the chemotherapy after breast cancer. I needed to lose weight, eat right, and strengthen my natural immunity in order to recover my health.

The entirety of what follows was researched and written by Abby regarding her experience with detoxification and nutrition prior to her own diagnosis with breast cancer in 2017. You can learn more about Abby Kurth at AbbyKurthNutrition. Coach (https://knowaboutnutrition.com/)

A Clinical Nutrition Approach to Recovery by Abby Kurth

Detoxification is definitely a topic for our times. Breast implant or no breast implant, people experiencing prolonged fatigue, digestive issues, mood changes, and the resulting frustration of undiagnosable symptoms is becoming a common phenomenon in our modern society despite (or in some circumstances because of) advances in medical technology.

I have never had a breast implant, but I have experienced the frustration of an undiagnosable condition. In 1986, I experienced a strange fever and pain in my liver over several days followed by a long-lasting fatigue and brain fog. This was before anyone had heard of chronic fatigue syndrome or the Epstein-Barr virus. After vowing to go to a doctor a day until I found out what was going on but still receiving no diagnosis after weeks, I realized it was up to me to find the answers. I studied nutrition, homeopathy, and functional medicine and worked on my various issues — yeast, hormone imbalance, and digestion. I kept myself going in this way.

After many years—I'm not proud to say it—I finally said to myself, "I shouldn't have to take all these supplements. If the zombie apocalypse comes, I'll be in trouble because I won't be able to find supplements to keep me functioning." Yes, I actually said that to myself. So, I stopped. Like a lobster in pot of water that is gradually warming up, I didn't pay attention to how awful I felt over the next few years.

My wake-up came when I realized my body could not relax, and my emotions were flat and I had no joy. Testing of the level of neurotransmitters, chemicals in the body that impact emotions, showed that I was low in serotonin, a calming neurotransmitter, and high in neurotransmitters that excite the nervous system. I began taking nutrients that increased the calming neurotransmitters. A diagnosis of breast cancer in 2017 really got my attention. I became a patient of a neurologist who looked at my genetics and worked on reducing inflammation, balancing the immune system, and supporting my thyroid. We also discovered a genetic defect for a metabolic pathway that increased the excitatory neurotransmitters causing the increased muscle tension, and I began using nutrients that improved this pathway. I began a regimen to eliminate bacterial overgrowth in the small intestine (small intestinal bacterial overgrowth or SIBO) and I was able to resolve that issue.

I now faithfully take my supplements and intravenous nutrients, and no zombie is going to stop me because I feel better than I have for a long, long time.

HELP FOR YOU

Hopefully, my story has helped people recognize that there is help for anyone. Everyone is different in their ability to access help, whether geographical or financial, so the ideal course of action for testing and obtaining professional help will be mentioned, but other self-help approaches will be given as well. Detoxification will be discussed, as that is an important part of healing due to the toxic nature of breast implants. Individual reaction may vary, but implants may also result in inflammation, immune reactions, mood changes, and/or overgrowth of unhealthy bacteria and fungi like yeast, so those topics will be discussed as a general health and nutrition pathway to healing.

People might need a realistic idea of what to expect for improvement, which is that it may take one month for every year they have been sick. Some sources have found it may take one to two years to recover health from breast implant illness. Healing will not happen overnight, but it will happen. Some women may find they need to go very slowly and/or that they make progress and then have a bad period for a time.

The good news is that there are more and more practitioners who recognize the need to treat the underlying cause of physical issues to be able to reverse chronic diseases. This area of medicine has been called Functional Medicine because the goal is to improve function of the body by removing what is harming the body (toxins, heavy metals, allergens, organisms like bacteria or yeast Candida albicans), and adds in what is missing (nutrients, probiotics, hormones).

One source for finding a Functional Medicine practitioner to help treat the impact of breast implants is the Institute for Functional Medicine (IFM.org). Licensed practitioners (MDs, D.O.s, dentists, pharmacists, nurses, chiropractors, registered dietitians, nurse practitioners, physician's assistants) can seek certification through this organization and be placed on the directory. Other practitioners with professional certifications like Certified Clinical Nutritionists (CCNs) (IAACN.org), or C.N.Cs (The American Association of Nutritional Consultants) have training in getting to the root cause of illness as well. Professional grade supplement companies hold training for the practitioners that use their products, and those companies may have a directory of knowledgeable professionals available to the public.

A well-trained professional is the ideal partner when undertaking detoxification. Functional medicine practitioners generally advise waiting approximately six months after surgery, or until digestion and elimination is working well before proceeding with detoxification. Once the individual's unique biochemistry and symptoms are known through functional testing (discussed later in this chapter), a professional can prepare a specially tailored detoxification program.

DETOXIFICATION IN THE BODY

Detoxification can be a big topic that can include any substance that can harm the body from the outside (food, water, air, chemicals) or the inside (implants, organisms). However, this information will focus most on the issues related to implants.

A person's susceptibility and response to toxins, in "varies by age, gender, genetic factors, nutritional status, other diseases, exposure pattern, and behavioral, lifestyle factors" as outlined in the book *Natural Detoxification: The Complete Guide to Clearing Your Body of Toxins* by Dr. Jacqueline Krohn, MD. Additionally, acid-alkaline balance in the body must be in an optimal range for detox pathways to function properly. Thus, each individual may be unique in their path to detoxification, as well as having unique needs because of the potential source of their toxins, breast implants.

Toxic exposure can interrupt the hundreds of biochemical reactions that take place in our body each second. Detoxification is such an important function that the body is designed so that any food eaten is taken immediately to the liver, the main organ of detoxification, to remove any harmful substances. Other organs supporting detoxification are skin, lungs, kidneys, bowels, and to a lesser degree, hair, sweat, and fingernails/toenails.

Detoxification has the potential of making a person feel worse, so it is wise to go slowly and gradually build up doses of the supporting supplements. Some supplements (chlorella, alpha-lipoic acid [ALA] or n-acetyl cysteine [NAC]) may mobilize mercury from dental fillings so a professional should be consulted before attempting detoxification.

LIVER

Detoxification in the liver happens in three phases. It is like gathering your trash, putting your trash in the bag, and taking your trash to the curb. Of course, one also needs to hope that the garbage man will take the trash away (and quickly!), which is what having regular bowel movements will accomplish.

The liver is the main organ of detoxification and it can store toxins for months, even years. In addition to toxins, the liver also metabolizes hormones and medications, and filters the blood from foreign debris, bacteria, and other waste. Here are some indications that the liver is overworked or poorly functioning: poor digestion, gas, constipation, loss of appetite, feeling of fullness, pain in the liver area (under right rib cage), nausea or pain after a fatty meal, headache, skin problems like acne or psoriasis, and moodiness or irritability.

Liver Detoxification Steps

Phase 0 — Toxins are imported into liver or kidney.

Phase 1 — Transformation: In this phase toxic compounds are rendered more water-soluble. These intermediates can be more toxic than the original compounds, especially if phase 2 is slow due to genetics or nutrition. These detoxification steps are also available in other organs and in the skin, but the liver is the real hero here. Some supporting supplements for this phase are nutrients (alpha-ketoglutaric acid, choline, fatty acids, lecithin, and thiamin (B-1), vitamins C and E, beta-carotene, iron, magnesium, manganese, zinc, sulphur, and molybdenum), amino acids (methionine) and the herb milk thistle. UltraClear Plus® pH from Metagenics is formulated to provide advanced, specialized support for balanced metabolic detoxification, including macronutrients (protein, carbohydrate, and fat) and micronutrients (vitamins, minerals, phytonutrients) to address liver function.

Phase 2 — Conjugation: Chemical groups are added (conjugated) to make the toxin able to be excreted through the bowel and kidney. The co-factors needed in this phase include nutrients (thiamine [B-1], riboflavin [B-2], niacin [B-3], pyridoxine [B-6] known in its active form as pyridoxal-5-phosphate, and vitamin B-12 as methylcobalamin ideally, and amino acids that come from proteins (glutamine, glycine, and cysteine). Sulphur foods such as broccoli, garlic, onions, and cauliflower are helpful as they help support the production of L-glutathione, an important detoxifying compound.

Some people may have a genetic mutation that creates difficulties with the MTHFR gene and methylation activity during Phase 2 liver detoxification. "The term methylation describes a biochemical process that is utilized in the body for transport of nutrients, energy production and in gene modulation. In patients with decreased methylation activity (i.e. methylation deficiency), there are significant shortcomings in the ability to execute a variety of important chemical functions in the body. These shortcomings can leave the body unprotected from the everyday assault of environmental and infectious agents, sluggish in neurotransmitter production, and slow to recover." per Dr. Kendall Stewart at GX Sciences[9]. Methylated forms of certain vitamins can overcome this genetic deficiency and improve the process.

Other sources writing on breast implant illness also mention the importance of methylation and the MTHFR gene. Discussions on breast implant illness cite information provided by Dr. Ben Lynch, "Dirty Genes: A Breakthrough Program to Treat the Root Cause of Illness and Optimize Your Health"), Amy Yasko (mthfr. dnatest.info, "Feel Good About Your SNPS"), and Dr. Lu-Jean Feng (You Tube). For further information, there are a series of podcasts, *Coffee with Dr. Stewart*, on neurobiologix.com including a podcast on MTHFR.

Phase 2.5 — Bile: This extra phase was added because so many people have issues with the gallbladder — think how many people we all know who have had their gallbladder removed! Bile is formed in the liver and stored in the gallbladder to be released when food is eaten so fats can be processed and absorbed. Bile does to the fats we eat what dish soap does to a greasy plate; it makes the grease water-soluble.

It is important to correct this process (and also the flow of lymph through the lymphatic system) before pushing detox. Coffee enemas help move bile and speed up the emptying of the bowel. There is a special circulatory system between the liver and the end of the colon called the enterohepatic circulation system. When the stool reaches this part of the bowel it is full of toxins and the coffee enema helps "get the trash out" quickly. The coffee enema also stimulates glutathione S-transferase, an enzyme which makes the liver detox pathways function. Helpful nutrients for this phase include: herbs (curcumin, artichoke, any bitter herb), amino acids (taurine, glycine), and phytonutrients (quercetin).

Phase 3 — Final conjugated toxins from the bile to excretion. Phase 3 is about transportation. It mainly refers to the transport of phase 2 conjugates either to the kidneys for further filtration and then out of the body via the bladder and urine, or out with bile into the small intestine, and down through the GI tract for elimination via stool. The key in this phase is to not let toxins be reabsorbed into the liver by the previously mentioned enterohepatic circulation cycle.

Helpful binders to prevent reabsorption of toxins include: bentonite clay, psyllium, activated charcoal, and zeolite. It is very important these binders be used away from food as they can prevent the absorption of food. The enterohepatic circulation cycle can also reabsorb estrogen that has been packaged by the liver to be removed in the stool but has been "unbound" by unhealthy bacteria in the gut and allowed to be taken back into the body. This contributes to hormonal imbalances.

DETOXIFICATION OF THE KIDNEY

There is support for helping the kidneys clear toxic waste. These include: herbs (artichoke, curcumin, stinging nettle, Cordyceps mushrooms, dandelion, grape seed, and green drinks to alkalinize the body), nutrients (phosphatidylcholine, N-acetyl cysteine [NAC], magnesium) and the hormone melatonin, which is available in supplement form.

CELLULAR DETOXIFICATION

Autophagy is the term that describes how the cell takes dead and decaying parts of the cells (organelles) and chews them up to be removed from the cell. When immune challenges and inflammation are present, the cell is not able to perform this function of repair and recovery.

There are ways to improve this process and allow the cells to repair, which is most important for cells in the immune and nervous system where prolonging the health of the cell greatly impacts life. Autophagy is greatly improved when inflammation is decreased, and anti-inflammatory support is provided by components in plants (curcumin, polyphenols, catechins, pycnogenol, resveratrol, quercetin), omega-3 fatty acids from flax and fish (EPA/DHA), vitamin C, and the prescription drug rapamycin.

Coenzyme Q10 is a supplement (ubiquinol is preferred form) that helps the cell's energy producing mitochondria. Any person on statin drugs for lowering cholesterol may be deficient in this nutrient because statins create a CoQ10 deficiency and the results are sometimes debilitating muscle cramps and weakness.

HOW TO DETOXIFY

Some people think detoxification is the same as a colon cleanse, thus the use of products along the lines of Colon Blow (yes, a real thing!). As can be seen, although moving waste through the colon is important, the steps that come before that are crucial as well. Also, people think that the worse they feel means they are doing a great job of detoxifying. Actually, they may really be increasing toxic intermediates and/or creating oxidative stress and damage. This process should be approached gently and by providing nutrient support to help the process along.

Other Detoxification Methods

Saunas or hot baths. Because toxins and heavy metals are often stored in the fat tissue, therapies that utilize heat are recommended to mobilize the toxins for elimination by the liver, kidney, and digestive tract. Infrared sauna is the ideal because it provides not only sweating, but also the added benefit of inducing cells to detoxify. Best results come when increasing circulation beforehand with exercise and washing off the toxins after the sauna with soap to prevent reabsorption per Dr. Dietrich Klinghardt of the Sophia Health Institute.[10]

Epsom salt baths. Magnesium sulfate, the primary mineral in Epsom salts, has a relaxing effect on muscles and the nervous system, reduces pain and inflammation, and the sulfate boosts the detoxification capabilities of both the skin and the liver. Sulfate draws out toxins through the skin and cleanses the liver by enhancing the production of bile. Hot baths with 1/2 cup (0.12 liters) of Epsom salts can be utilized for ten to twenty minutes three times a day.

Oxygen Therapy: Ozone is an unstable oxygen molecule that can be found in nature or created. Bacteria and viruses can be cleansed from the blood with ozone at special infusion centers that withdraw blood, treat it with ozone, and replace it into the body. Ozone also has anti-tumor properties.

Oxygen Therapy: Hyperbaric oxygen therapy is oxygen administered under pressure to increase the oxygenation of the blood. This is done in a special hyperbaric oxygen chamber and the process can cleanse the body of microorganisms.

Oxygen Therapy: Hydrogen peroxide occurs in nature and is created in the body as part of the immune defense. Dr. Jacqueline Krohn, in *Natural Detoxification: The Complete Guide to Clearing Your Body of Toxins,* offers specific instructions for using hydrogen peroxide. Always follow hydrogen peroxide treatment with probiotic replacement.

Homeopathy. Many people think the term homeopathy is the whole realm of natural medicine, but actually homeopathy is a specific system of treatment that was advanced by physician Samuel Hahnemann over 200 years ago. The main philosophy of homeopathy is that "like cures like" and trained practitioners will know how to match physical, mental, and emotional symptoms with a specially prepared remedy from natural substances. That being said, generally, using low potency remedies (6x, 12x, 30x, 30c) like silica and platina (platinum) for the main toxic metals in implants will do no harm (classical homeopaths may cringe at this). The one exception would be that homeopathic silica has a reputation for being good at stimulating the elimination of foreign bodies and so should only be used after implants have been removed. Nux vomica is a general remedy that is helpful for detoxification. If the remedies don't work, it may be because the correct remedy isn't being used. Some homeopaths are trained in detoxification techniques and the National Center for Homeopathy can be a resource for finding those practitioners.

GENERAL HEALTH AND NUTRITION

Surprise (or no surprise), but not everything on the Internet is accurate. The references provided here do offer sound advice. Almost every practitioner will have his or her own opinions on the matter, which, unfortunately, can be confusing. The recommendations here are a compilation from several practitioners and from professional conferences.

One benefit of contacting a professional to help guide the healing process is that tests can be ordered to find each person's unique issues. We are all truly individual and how we get sick and what we need to get better can vary from person to person. Here are some tests that can be helpful in guiding return to health.

Genetic testing can determine weaknesses in the metabolic pathways that lead to inflammation, abnormal immune response, detoxification, genetic issues with neurotransmitters (the brain chemicals that impact mood). GXSciences.com and Genova Diagnostics Laboratory are two sources for identifying the genes that can be modified to improve health. Not every genetic test on the market these days looks at the genes that are actually useful to improve health.

Heavy metal testing can identify what toxic metals are being retained in the body. Genova Diagnostics Laboratory (gdx.net) offers several tests including the Toxic Element Clearance Profile, which measures toxic metals in the urine before and after administration of a chelating agent given to bind metals.

Nutrient deficiencies. If nutrients are deficient, the body cannot perform any function including immunity, detoxification, repair and recovery, and growth. Additionally, being deficient in healthy minerals may allow the body to take up toxic minerals (lead, arsenic, mercury). Knowing specifically what nutrients are deficient can allow individualized supplementation. Some vitamin and mineral levels can be measured through blood. A specialized test, Cellular Nutrition, is offered by SpectraCell Laboratories (spectracell.com). Genova offers ONE (Optimal Nutritional Evaluation) testing.

Neurotransmitter Testing

Neurotransmitters are chemicals that communicate information throughout your brain and body. They relay information between neuron to neuron and tell your heart to beat, lungs to breath, and stomach to digest. Neurotransmitter testing would be helpful for people experiencing poor sleep, ADD/ADHD, anxiety, depression, memory issues, and more. ZRT Laboratory is one lab that offers neurotransmitter testing.

Harmful organisms

Tests such as the Genova GI Effects Comprehensive Profile from stool can identify bacteria, fungus (yeast), and parasites that may be part of the root cause of illness. This test will identify the exact prescription or herbal product that will kill a person's specific organism as not everyone responds to the same therapeutic approach.

Breath tests, which capture exhaled hydrogen (H2) and methane (CH4) gases after a patient drinks a lactulose sugar solution, are used to test for organisms growing in the small bowel (SIBO). The Genova Small Intestine Bacterial Overgrowth test showed positive where my doctor's test showed negative for me, because it has the added benefit of looking for both hydrogen and methane. This test has people follow a special diet before testing to get a true baseline level.

Immune System

Immunoglobulins (Ig), also known as antibodies, act as a critical part of the immune response by recognizing, binding to, and helping destroy foreign invaders like bacteria, fungus, or viruses. Immunoglobulin E (IgE) level may be higher in the blood serum level of women with silicone breast implants because the body's immune system feels there is an immediate threat.

Silicone acts as an adjuvant, which is a substance that provides constant nonspecific stimulation of the immune system. Adjuvants, like alumina, are added to vaccinations to keep the immune system stimulated, so care should be taken if implants are already creating immune overstimulation. There are currently two medical tests for silicone in the body, the silicone antibody test and a blood level for silicon.

Because the immune system is triggered by silicone implants, food, food additives, and environmental chemicals can further trigger the immune system to launch into action, creating all those symptoms we associate with allergy and immune over-activation. Traditional food allergy testing (RAST, skin tests) looks for IgE and immediate allergic reactions. Other labs will also test for Immunoglobulin G (IgG) and/or observe changes in cells that might show a more delayed allergic reaction to various foods not picked up on a RAST test. The IgG antibodies may have a delayed hypersensitivity reaction which is more subtle than the immediate reaction, ranging from gastrointestinal bloating and nausea to headaches, mood changes, and fatigue. Because they occur long after eating an "offending" food, the symptoms might not be recognized as being due to that food.

Endocrine system

Blood, urine, or saliva can be tested to look at hormone levels for estrogen and progesterone. Estrogen causes cells to proliferate or multiply and so is pro-cancer, while progesterone puts the brakes on cell multiplication and is anti-cancer. Excess estrogen also impacts detoxification through the liver and bile. I wish I had paid more attention to the lack of progesterone compared to estrogen (proliferation index) on the salivary hormone testing I had, and I might have avoided a breast tumor. Genetic testing also showed that I had an issue with clearing estrogen from my body.

Other endocrine problems seen in breast implant illness might be issues with the adrenal gland and the health of the adrenal gland can be determined with a twenty-four-hour salivary cortisol test. The thyroid gland may also be impacted and a thorough thyroid evaluation would include free T3, free T4, reverse T3, and possibly some testing for thyroid antibodies.

Organic Acid Testing

Organic acid testing is sort of the pot luck of testing. By looking at waste products of metabolism in the urine, a test like the Organix® Comprehensive Nutritional Test, or organic acid testing in general, is valuable for determining many conditions such as functional vitamin and mineral status, amino acid deficiencies, oxidative damage, phase 1 and 2 detoxification capacity, functional B-complex vitamin need, neurotransmitter metabolites, methylation issues, and markers for bacterial and yeast overgrowth.

PATHWAY TO HEALING

The formula for anyone seeking to overcome chronically poor health, breast implants or not, is the same: Remove what is harming, replace what is missing, heal the gut, and balance the immune system. Individuals may vary in what damage has occurred from breast implants or their body's needs but addressing these needs will provide the ability for healing to take place.

Step #1: REMOVE WHAT IS HARMING

(One to two months pre-surgery then continue)

Beginning to remove the burdens on the body from toxins, immune challenges, stress, and inflammation is the place to start, especially if preparing for explant surgery.

IMPLANTS. Breast implants impact the immune and endocrine systems. Implants create an environment conducive to harmful organisms, impact detoxification, and are highly inflammatory to tissues, organs, and glands. That is why removing the implants is important, but it is wise to prepare for surgery by working on the first two steps until health is somewhat improved.

INFLAMMATORY FOODS. Everything our body does—fight illness, detoxify, repair, growth, or immunity—is done with the nutrients we get from our food. Our body doesn't run on medications or man-made food; it runs on food as it comes in nature. Period.

Processed or "non" foods offer little nutrition and are often inflammatory. Some people have found weight loss and renewed health just limiting themselves to foods that have five or fewer ingredients on the label. The reason? These foods likely have less sugar, dyes, and/or preservatives and may contain more fiber and nutrients.

Ultra-processed foods like packaged breads and pastries, frozen pizzas and chicken nuggets, sodas, and potato chips contain substances made in laboratories, have had healthy ingredients taken away (fiber, vitamins, and minerals) and have ingredients not seen in nature added (high fructose corn syrup, hydrogenated oils). These processed foods are designed to be addictive. The body responds well when we remove these foods from our diet.

HARMFUL ORGANISMS. Another thing these harmful non-foods do is feed the unhealthy organisms in our digestive tract. The human microbiome is the collection of trillions of microbes living in and on the human body. Researchers of the Microbiome Project are studying the organisms in our digestive tract and finding how they contribute to either health or disease. One important finding of the microbiome is that it changes in response to what food is eaten.

Diets high in processed foods favor the growth of organisms that are not helpful or healthful such as yeast, bacteria, and parasites. These organisms put out their own waste, which our body has to detoxify, and they also trigger our immune system to respond over a long period of time.

Breast implant illness often includes overgrowth of yeast (candidiasis) and may lead to symptoms such as fatigue, muscle aches, diarrhea, abdominal cramps, memory loss, vaginal yeast infections, and bloating. Yeast is hard to get rid of. A medical practitioner may need to prescribe Diflucan and/or Nystatin. Some natural products people have used are Yeast Connection, Harmon Formulas Candida Program, Candistroy by Nature's Secret, Biocidin protocol, oil of oregano, and garlic.

I used the Biocidin protocol for six months to finally get rid of the organisms that were bothering me as other shorter attempts did not solve the problem. How effective the previously mentioned products might be varied from person to person, thus the recommendation for testing before starting an attempt to get rid of these harmful organisms. To avoid the microbe from developing a tolerance, it is often recommended rotating the product used. An Anti-Candida/Low Mycotoxin diet will starve the organisms, which is another reason to ditch the added sugars and refined carbs.

People can feel worse when they start to kill off these organisms. This is called the Herxheimer reaction. The Herxheimer Reaction is a short-term (from days to a few weeks) detoxification reaction in the body because the dying organisms are putting out byproducts like acetaldehyde. It is not uncommon to experience flu-like symptoms including headache, joint and muscle pain, body aches, sore throat, general malaise, sweating, chills, nausea, brain fog, irritability, bloating, diarrhea or constipation, joint pain, or other symptoms. Taking activated charcoal at different times from ingesting medications and food (activated charcoal affects absorption) is helpful for avoiding Herxheimer symptoms. Vitamin C and molybdenum are also helpful.

IMMUNE REACTIVE FOODS. Some foods trigger an immune reaction for people. Again, these reactions are individual and can be determined by testing as previously discussed. The most common offending foods are eggs, milk, peanuts, tree nuts, fish, shellfish, wheat, soy.[11]

Some sources that write about breast implant illness recommend eliminating nightshade vegetables. Nightshade vegetables are tomatoes, potatoes (but not sweet potatoes), eggplant, bell peppers, spices sourced from peppers, such as cayenne and paprika. That doesn't mean everyone should be cutting these nutritious foods from their diet, according to the Cleveland Clinic article "What's the Deal with Nightshade Vegetables?"

According to the author of this article, "A food sensitivity is very patient-specific and can often be a symptom of another imbalance rather than a permanent problem with that food." However, if a trial elimination of the food shows benefit, then elimination should be considered, especially if other inflammatory conditions like arthritis, inflammatory bowel disease, or psoriasis are present.

STRESS. Psychological and physiological stress can put us into a state where the sympathetic nervous system (fight or flight) predominates. Fight or flight is how the body prepares when it sees a stressor (lion or bear) or imagines a stressor ("My boss doesn't like me"). Calming inflammation and making the body more alkaline can help push the body toward the parasympathetic nervous system, which is where digestion and repair can take place. Psychological techniques such as prayer, meditation, and gratitude help this process as well. Being kind to one's self is helpful in the healing process.

HOW TO CHANGE HARMFUL HABITS. So how does one begin to make these changes? Here are some thoughts: 1. Try the "5 ingredients or fewer" rule when shopping outside the fresh meats and produce aisles. 2. Reduce or substitut processed, inflammatory "non" foods for a healthy food. 3. Find a food list base on the Mediterranean diet and plan to incorporate more of those foods. 4. If yo lack confidence or feel overwhelmed, I have a book entitled *Sick and Tired, t Healthy and Inspired: 9 Steps to Prevent Lifestyle Related Diseases* that make it easy for people to make changes in healthy eating and exercise available o Amazon (https://www.amazon.com/author/nutritioncoachabbykurth) or o abbykurthnutrition.coach (https://knowaboutnutrition.com/shop/).

Step #2: ADD WHAT IS NEEDED
(One to two months pre-surgery then continue)

This step involves adding back what the body is lacking. In our modern society, we often don't get quality whole foods, probiotics, nutrients, water, or movement, and this can result in hormone imbalances.

WHOLE FOODS

So much in the body will begin to repair itself when it is getting the right fuel — whole foods. I have worked with the Mediterranean Diet, which is well-researche for being anti-inflammatory as well as anti-cancer, anti-diabetes, and anti-hear disease.

The backbone of the Mediterranean Diet includes:

- Healthy fats from olive oil, fish, avocados, and nuts
- Lots of vegetables, including both cruciferous and green leafy vegetables such as broccoli, spinach, and kale. Eating some raw fruits and vegetables daily is ideal.
- Lots of fresh fruits, especially melons and berries that have less impact or blood sugar
- Whole grains and legumes that are naturally high in fiber
- Meat is used in small portion sizes (4–6 ounces). Organic, wild, free-range, or pasture raised are ideal.

Based on cell health testing (bioimpedance) one can watch the improvemen in clients who follow this whole food diet closely. These whole foods are high i antioxidants to curb oxidative stress, are anti-inflammatory, and have fiber, whic nourishes beneficial organisms in the gut and balances blood sugar.

High plant-based diets are also alkaline instead of acidic because of their hig mineral content. This supports the part of the nervous system (parasympathetic that helps repair and recovery of the body, and harmful organisms (yeast, bacteria) cannot grow when the body is alkaline (over 7.4 pH). When the body is receiving the minerals it needs, it is less likely to hold on to toxic minerals like mercury, lead, or the toxic minerals in breast implants.

The Gerson Therapy diet, which reports success, is used frequently for patients with cancer. Those who have autoimmune symptoms can follow the Paleo Autoimmune Protocol diet to reduce inflammation in the gut. If the gut is greatly compromised, people may need to start with the GAPS (Gut and Psychology Syndrome) by Dr. Natasha Campbell-McBride, or the Specific Carbohydrate Diet by Elaine Gottschall.[12]

One often recommended gut health food is bone broth, which is made by simmering bones over a period of time. This simmering causes the bones and ligaments to release healing compounds like collagen, proline, glycine, and glutamine that have the power to transform health.

Ideally, the foods you eat should be organic when possible. One doctor tells a story of a businessman who resisted using the scruffy looking organic carrot to juice but noticed a marked improvement in how he felt when using organic carrots instead of non-organic. Recently we have seen food "manufacturers" developing genetically modified (GMO) foods, which are designed to tolerate greater levels of pesticides by introducing engineered viruses or bacteria into the plants' genetic code. Unfortunately, these engineered organisms are seen as a foreign invader and can be an immune trigger for many people.

All vegetables, fruits, and even eggs and meats can be washed well with something like lemon, vinegar, or sea salt saltwater to kill any organisms. There are also commercial vegetable washes available.

Plants rock. We are beginning to discover the benefit of the phytonutrients contained in plants and even our common kitchen herbs contain many benefits. Green tea, turmeric or curcumin, ginger and rosemary are all antioxidant and anti-inflammatory.

PROBIOTICS. The word *probiotic* means "for life," and probiotics are foods or supplements that contain the healthy bacteria that promote a healthy life and a healthy microbiome. If taking a probiotic supplement, a good probiotic should:

- Have as many species of beneficial bacterial as possible.
- Ideally have a combination of lactobacilli, bifidobacteria, and soil bacteria.
- Contain as many bacteria as possible, at least eight billion bacteria per gram.
- Be tested and manufacturer should be monitored by a third party for quality.

- Saccharomyces boulardii is an organism that seems to be helpful in combating the yeast infections caused by Candida albicans.

Probiotics may need to be gradually introduced and increased, staying at the same dose if there is a "die-off reaction" and then continuing to increase as the person's system allows. It may take a few weeks to a few months to reach a therapeutic dose, which Dr. Campbell-McBride, author of *Gut and Psychology Syndrome* indicates is around 15–20 billion of bacterial cells per day for an adult. The therapeutic dose should be continued for six months and then can be reduced to a maintenance dose level.

Fermented foods are readily available at health food stores (tea, pickles, sauerkraut, kimchi, miso, yogurt, kefir, and kombucha), or can be made at home (search for Dr. Joseph Mercola's Cultured Vegetables Recipe).

Some people with digestive issues might find more bloating with probiotic formulas that also contain prebiotics, which are non-digestible, fermentable fibers from food that help feed the probiotic organisms. The bottle might show as the ingredient substances like inulin, Fructo-oligosaccharides (FOS), arabinogalactans or chicory root. Prebiotics like these are normally helpful, but people with yeast issues might find prebiotics cause more gas than desired.

TARGETED SUPPLEMENTS. The *right* supplements in the *right* amount for the *right* indication for the right individual at the *right* time.

I have seen people come for appointments with a whole grocery bag filled with supplements they have read about and decided they needed. Unfortunately, these people are not necessarily feeling better and may actually be feeling worse. Firstly, without specific testing, there is no proof they actually need these supplements. Secondly, some may be buying poor quality supplements that aren't in a form that can be used (for example, people with poor MTHR gene function would do best with methylated B vitamins). Finally, too much too soon can overwhelm the body before it is able to absorb and use these supplements.

As a self-confessed person who doesn't like to take too many supplements, I find that it works best to limit to four to six supplement products that are designed to support a specific function (immune support, detoxification, antioxidant, anti-inflammatory), contain a combination of nutrients for that particular function (one pill contains all the nutrients or herbs that work together synergistically), are indicated based on individualized testing, are introduced at the appropriate time in the healing process, and do not contain binders, dyes, fillers.

If possible, supplements should be gluten free, soy free, yeast free, sugar free, preservative free, and anything else one may need to avoid based on personal allergies. Pharmaceutical grade silicon dioxide (silica), often used in supplements, caused eighteen times the immune reaction for women who had implants and should be avoided if at all possible based on the recommendations of Dr. Shanklin, Dr. Smalley, et al. in the article "Immunologic Stimulation of T Lymphocytes by Silica After Use of Silicone Mammary Implants."[13] Ideally supplements should also be monitored for quality by an independent third party and given a seal of quality from groups like ConsumerLab.com, NSF International, and U.S. Pharmacopeia (USP).

WATER. The ideal source of water would be spring water that contains natural forms of minerals. If this is not available or practical, reverse osmosis water will have contaminants removed, and there are products available to add minerals back into the water. If tap water is all that is available, it can be left out for twenty minutes to allow the chlorine to evaporate. Recommendations are for eight glasses of eight ounces each, or half the body weight in ounces per day.

HORMONES. Melatonin for sleep is the only hormone I would recommend people take without functional testing. Ideally, a practitioner would prescribe bio-identical hormones to replace/balance estrogen, progesterone, DHEA, and testosterone after hormone testing. Functional practitioners often prefer natural porcine (NP) thyroid medication, as it is a natural hormone versus a synthetic preparation.

MOVEMENT. Gentle exercise will keep up circulation of lymph, blood, and oxygen. For example, a thirty-minute walk three times a week and two days of yoga or gentle stretching would provide support without overwhelming the body as it heals.

HOW TO START

How to begin adding in healing foods? Consider joining a Facebook group for the Mediterranean diet, enrolling in e-meals.com to find recipes, or search online for "healthy, quick meals." Small goals work best, so setting a goal to try two new whole foods each week will help make progress. Similarly, set an easy beginning exercise goal. Begin to research a functional practitioner that can help develop a supplement and hormone plan.

STEP #3: HEAL THE GUT
(Continue for possibly six months or more)

Most functional professionals have been taught the four Rs of healing the gut: remove, reinocculate, replace, and repair. This is an important part of the healing process as unhealthy organisms in the intestinal tract and ongoing inflammation can impact digestion and absorption of food and nutrients, worsening an already bad situation. Additionally, it has been discovered that there is a gut-brain connection, so poor gut health and gut organisms can lead to changes in the brain and vice versa. Anxiety and depression are now being recognized as a result of the impact of the microbiome on mood related neurotransmitters. Here are the steps to improve gut health.

1. **Remove.** This includes allergenic foods and pathogenic organisms as discussed in Step #1.

2. **Reinocculate.** Adding in probiotics and prebiotics as discussed in Step #2.

3. **Replace.** When the digestion process is healthy, hydrochloric acid (HCL) is secreted to begin the digestion process in the stomach, and this acid triggers the release of digestive enzymes by the pancreas to break down proteins (protease), fats (lipase), and starch (amylase). Lab tests such as fat absorption tests and gastric analysis can help determine what factors may need to be replaced.

Lack of stomach acid or hypochlorhydria worsens with aging. Oftentimes when someone has hyperacidity after a meal, it might interestingly be a sign the stomach actually needs more acid to digest. People can try one tablespoon of fresh lemon juice with eight ounces of water about twenty minutes before a meal. If symptoms worsen instead of improve, then this should be discontinued, but if symptoms improve that means the extra acid is helping and the lemon water can be continued to support digestion. Betaine HCL is also a supplement to replace stomach acid.

Easily breaking fingernails can be a sign of low stomach acid because minerals must be dissolved by acid for them to be absorbed and used in the body. Other signs of low stomach acid can be bloating, burping, diarrhea, gas, and/or hair loss. This lack of acid sets up the possibility of pathogens (bacteria, yeast, parasites) inhabiting the lower intestinal tract, as they are not killed in the stomach.

Lack of digestive enzymes from the pancreas may present as stools that are fatty, pale, bulky, bad smelling, and difficult to flush, as well as diarrhea, stomach pain, gas and bloating, and/or vitamin deficiency. Both stomach acid and bile trigger the release of pancreatic enzymes so improving those processes will help, but supplementation may still be necessary. A helpful supplement to replace digestive enzymes should include lipase, protease, and amylase. If special help is needed with gluten, the DPP IV enzyme may be included, though avoidance of gluten is the preference to avoid inflaming the intestinal lining.

4. **Repair.** The Leaky Gut Syndrome involves weakening of the tight junctions between cells in the small intestine where absorption of nutrients takes place.

Normally this junction lets in small size molecules of digested food, somewhat like the airport security line. Imagine if the waiting passengers overran the security checkpoint — this is leaky gut. These loose or "leaky" connections allow larger particles of food to cross the intestinal barrier than would normally be likely, and these particles trigger the immune system because they appear to be foreign invaders. The previous symptoms (bloating, gas) plus fatigue, headache, and joint pain can result.

STEP #4: BALANCE IMMUNE SYSTEM

All of the previous steps will have lessened the burden on the immune system by removing the things that excite or up-regulate immune response — unhealthy intestinal organisms and breast implants. There are a few more things that can help the immune system.

Oxidation is a process that creates components (free radicals) that can damage cells. Antioxidants are the heroes that stop this process. Antioxidants can be obtained through foods or supplements that are high in beta-carotene, vitamin E, selenium, vitamin C, and coenzyme Q10 (CoQ10), which also helps with cell energy.

Colostrum is the first milk after giving birth that is high in antibodies. Most supplements obtain this from cows, and this can provide the material to defend against viruses, bacteria, and parasites. Certain mushrooms, maitaki and shitaki to name two, have undigestible carbohydrate called beta-glucans. Ongoing research suggests that beta-glucans can trigger many different types of immune cells to begin to do their work in the body.

NEVER GIVE UP

These four steps may feel totally overwhelming. Don't be discouraged. We all have to learn how to be our body's best friend and what we can do to help it heal. The body is an amazing machine that can repair and recover all the systems we have talked about —immune, digestion, detoxification, brain/nervous system, and endocrine (hormones). Any small change in lifestyle, or any small step towards support of healing, will allow the body to work to overcome the impact of implants. For more information contact abbykurthnutrition.coach.

Group Discussion Questions

1. Have you felt medical professionals and family and friends dismissed your concerns and symptoms? Have you ignored your changing health?
2. Who has supported you on your journey of breast implant illness?
3. What do you think you have lost during this experience? What have you gained?
4. When have you tried to find healing?
5. Why do you think the author included the information on spiritual and emotional healing?
6. Do you know what to do in order to achieve wholeness?
7. What are your next steps going to be?
8. How is the experience of breast cancer survivors with reconstruction different from the women with augmentation or enlargement surgeries? Is there any difference in seeking help for the illness?
9. What would you want to tell women considering breast implants for any reason?
10. How will you address this with your medical personnel?
11. Why do you think you decided to have reconstruction or augmentation?
12. How has the decision to have implants and/or explants affected your life? Positive? Negative? How has it impacted your relationships?

Endnotes

1   Source: Nikki Castel, Taylor Soon-Sutton, Peter Deptula, Anna Flaherty, and Fereydoun Don Parsa. https://www.ncbi.nlm.nih.gov/pmc/articles/ PMC4366700/ Archive Plastic Surgery 2015 Mar; 42(2): 186–193.Published online 2015 Mar 16. doi: 1. Ashley FL. A new type of breast prosthesis. Preliminary report. Plast Reconstr Surg. 1970;45:421–424. 2. U.S. Food and Drug Administration. FDA breast implant consumer handbook 2004: timeline of breast implant activities. Silver Spring, MD: U.S. Food and Drug Administration; 2013. 3. Van Zele D, Heymans O. Breast implants. A review. Acta Chir Belg. 2004;104:158–165.

2   Reflexology-research.com

3   Alternativesforhealing.com

4   Healingdaily.com

5   Bernie S. Siegel, M.D., Love, Medicine and Miracles 1st edition (New York: HarperCollins, 1986)

6   Edith Schaeffer, *The Tapestry: The Life and Times of Francis and Edith Schaeffer*, Special Memorial Edition November 1984, (Waco: Word Books,1981), 348, 615.

7   Shane Claiborne, Jonathan Wilson-Hartgrove, and Enuma Okoro, *Common Prayer: A Liturgy for Ordinary Radicals*, (Grand Rapids: Zondervan, 2010)

8   Surgery.org/TheAestheticsSociety/BreastImplantIllness/ Frequently Asked Questions and Talking Points/Updated 8/25/20

9   Stewart, Kendall. GXsciences.com. Foundation/Methylation/Wellness Panel, https://www.gxsciences.com/methylation-testing-s/2.htm. GX Sciences, Inc. 2020.

10   Dr. Dietrich Klinghardt of the Sophia Health Institute, "How to Maximize the Benefits of Sauna for Detoxification," The Great Plains Laboratory, Inc.

11   American College of Allergy, Allergy, and Immunology acaai.org

12   Natasha Campbell-McBride, MD, *Gut and Psychology Syndrome*, (White River Junction: Medinform Publishing, 2012).

13   DL Smalley, DR Shanklin, MF Hall, MV Stevens, and A Hanissian, "Immunologic Stimulation of T Lymphocytes by Silica After Use of Silicone Mammary Implants," FASEB J. 1995 March 9 (5): 424-7

Recommended Resources

Facebook (private groups you must request to join)
- https://Facebook.com/breastimplantillnesshealingwarriors 8,500 members
- https://Facebook.com/breastimplantillnessandbreastcancersurvivors 1,200 members
- Https://Facebook.com/breastimplantillnessjourneybacktohealth 4,300 members
- https://Facebook.com/breastimplantillnessawareness
- https://Facebook.com/breastimplantillnessandhealingbynicole 108,000 members
- https://Facebook.com/Breastimplantlawsuits 10,000 members
- https://www.facebook.com/Breast-implants-medical-case-reports-forensics-and-more-573210066074198
- https://www.facebook.com/breast_implant_illness_research_&_recovery, Inc. Group 5,400 members

Websites
- Https://healingbreastimplantillness.com
- My experience of Breast Implant Illness, *Medical News Today,* "Through my eyes: Breast implant illness"

Television
The Doctors, "Breast Implant Illness: Can Removal Reverse the Sickness?"

YouTube
Search Breast Implant Illness for many videos

Instagram
#breastimplantillness, over 49K posts
#breastimplantswereNEVERsafe

Bloggers
- https://reversingbreastimplantillness.com/
- www.biiaware.com

- http://www.dryoun.com/blog/what-you-need-to-know-about-breast-implant-illness-and-my-opinion-on-bii/

Podcasts
- Susan Liana Douglas
- Anthony William – Medical Medium
- Kitty Martone – Stuff your Doctor should Know
- Manifestationbabe.com
- The Chalene Show

Articles
- "What We Wished We Had Known About Boob Jobs"
- FDA MedWatch Voluntary Reporting Form or by calling 1-800-FDA-1088.
- https://www.fda.gov/medical-devices/breast-implants/risks-and-complications-breast-implants
- "Special Report: Breast Implant Illness and BIA-ALCL" (breast implant-associated anaplastic large cell lymphoma)

Payment by Insurance for Breast Cancer patients who want to Explant

- Breastcancer.org/Federal law — the Women's Health and Cancer Rights Act of 1998 — requires health insurance companies to pay for breast reconstruction surgeries if they pay for mastectomies. This includes covering all stages of reconstruction and treatment of any complications that result from a mastectomy or reconstruction.
- https://www.dol.gov/sites/dolgov/files/ebsa/about-ebsa/our-activities/resource-center/publications/your-rights-after-a-mastectomy.pdf
- MD Anderson Doctors issue breast implant warning – 9/24/18 https://www.necn.com/news/national-international/doctors-issue-breast-implant-warning/2092416/

Books
- *The Naked Truth about Breast Implants: From Harm to Healing,* Dr. Susan Kolb (as of 1/2020 she no longer has hospital privileges)
- Are Your Fake Boobs Making You Sick, Jen Herrera

- Quick Guide to Breast Implant Illness, Gloria Rose
- Let Me Get This Off My Chest: An inspiring story of saving my own life and my journey to self love, Tara Hopko
- Killer Breasts: Overcoming Breast Implant Illness, Diane Kazer FDN-P HHC
- She Fought on Her Knees: My Story with Breast Implant Illness, Angelia Russell
- Let Me Get This Off My Chest: A Breast Cancer Survivor Over-Shares, Margaret Lesh, Allyson Ryan, et al.